The
Hyperacusis and
Misophonia Book

The Hyperacusis and Misophonia Book

WHEN EVERYDAY SOUNDS ARE TOO LOUD, DISTRESSING, OR PAINFUL

James A. Henry

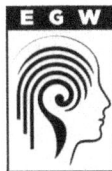

Ears Gone Wrong, LLC

978-1-962629-10-2 (paperback)

978-1-962629-11-9 (ebook)

978-1-962629-09-6 (hardback)

Contents

Foreword

The word hyperacusis originates from the Latin "hyper" (over) and "acusis" (hearing). While this term denoting "overhearing" may seem straightforward, classifying the variety of conditions diagnosed as "hyperacusis" is anything but uncomplicated, creating confusion for doctors and patients alike. One person might hear things louder while another might hear things painfully. Others might have emotional, rather than physical, responses to sound. Some cases represent merely an annoyance and inconvenience to daily life, while others are completely incapacitated—making the distinction not simply a quest for clarity of terminology, but of critical importance for research and patient management.

At last! Thanks to Dr. James Henry's *The Hyperacusis and Misophonia Book: When Everyday Sounds Are Too Loud, Distressing, or Painful*, we now have a superb resource. His book thoroughly addresses the complexities of these misunderstood medical conditions and provides a guide for patients, families, friends, doctors, and researchers.

As someone deeply involved in supporting hyperacusis patients through online patient support groups, I routinely see the confusion that surrounds sound hypersensitivity disorders. Every day, new patients join our groups, often overwhelmed and unsure of their symptoms and diagnosis. Longtime support group members do their best to provide guidance, but this ad hoc process has always lacked a definitive, comprehensive resource. Dr. Henry's book will be invaluable to educate and guide people.

One reason for patient confusion is unfamiliarity among providers. As a patient, I experienced this firsthand. For most of my life I had no sound hypersensitivity whatsoever. In fact, I loved loud noises—the US Navy Blue Angels air show with its screaming jet engines was a favorite. That all changed when I began to enter middle age, about 10 years ago, and sounds began to cause ear pain. I consulted with two leading specialists. They were uncertain about whether I had misophonia or hyperacusis. While it is clear to me now that I have loudness and pain hyperacusis, I wish the information presented in Dr. Henry's book had been available back then.

Clarifying a patient's type of sound hypersensitivity disorder is critical because approaches to managing the conditions vary dramatically. What can be helpful for one patient group may be actively harmful for another. In my own case, the suggested treatment was sound therapy. I followed this advice, but unfortunately it worsened me. What likely would have helped in my case was avoidance of sounds that were painful, which may have held my condition to a milder level. Instead, it progressed to a severe level, where it has remained.

This book is pivotal for medical researchers as well. As a volunteer with the nonprofit Hyperacusis Research, I raise money to fund research grants for hyperacusis, which are awarded to medical researchers through our partner Hearing Health Foundation. But these researchers are often no more clear on the different types of sound hypersensitivity disorders than are patients and providers. It is vital for researchers to understand the nuances of these disorders. The clear definitions and subtyping as laid out in Dr. Henry's book will allow researchers to focus their efforts in a manner that aligns with subtypes of patient symptoms, thereby accelerating progress and ultimately improving lives.

I look forward to recommending Dr. Henry's book to all of these audiences—patients, families, friends, doctors, and researchers. This book undoubtedly will help provide clarity for anyone affected by sound hypersensitivity disorders and those dedicated to understanding and treating them.

David Treworgy
Hyperacusis patient
Member, Board of Directors, Hyperacusis Research

Preface

This book focuses on what I refer to as *sound hypersensitivity disorders*. Although these disorders have always existed, the different types of disorders are still being distinguished, described, and named. Unfortunately, we are nowhere near reaching consensus, which is necessary to unify this young and emerging field.

Historically, *hyperacusis* has referred to any form of decreased tolerance to sound. Hyperacusis has been distinguished from misophonia fairly recently. There are actually *five* distinguishable sound hypersensitivity disorders: loudness hyperacusis, pain hyperacusis, misophonia, noise sensitivity, and phonophobia. This book describes each of them with respect to similarities, differences, and methods of clinical assessment, diagnosis, and treatment.

Personally, I have *loudness hyperacusis*—I don't have pain hyperacusis nor any of the other four sound hypersensitivity disorders. I also have hearing loss and tinnitus—all caused by loud music and carpentry during my younger years. Because of my loudness hyperacusis, I used to wear earplugs whenever I was outdoors or driving. I attended a training seminar for Tinnitus Retraining Therapy (TRT) where I realized that wearing earplugs was only making my loudness hyperacusis worse. I learned to gradually reduce the use of earplugs and to expose myself to safe levels of sound as much as possible—to *desensitize* my auditory system. Making those changes helped significantly, but I still have difficulty tolerating sound when it reaches a certain level. I carry custom-fit "musician" earplugs with me, and I use them whenever sound is uncomfortably loud. I *manage* my loudness hyperacusis, and it has a minimal effect on my life.

People with *pain hyperacusis* may not be so fortunate. Some of these people cannot tolerate sound *at all*. The advice I received at the TRT seminar would not normally work for a person with pain hyperacusis. This disorder can cause a person to continually wear earplugs and/or earmuffs whenever out in public, but also sometimes within their own homes. Fortunately, research is providing insights about pain hyperacusis and types of treatment that are available.

Whereas both forms of hyperacusis involve physical discomfort when exposed to sound, misophonia and noise sensitivity are characterized by *emotional reactions* to sound. With *misophonia*, the person reacts to *certain sounds* that usually come from the mouth or nose of other people. The reactions usually involve strong negative emotions. *Noise sensitivity* refers to hypersensitivity to sound *in general*, regardless of its source. People with noise sensitivity typically prefer to be in quiet or sound-controlled environments. Sound that reaches a certain level causes irritation/annoyance.

Phonophobia does not refer to reactions to sound but rather to *unhealthy fear* that sound will be uncomfortable for any reason. It is a *phobia* that is characterized by anxiety, and it can accompany one or more of the other sound hypersensitivity disorders. In fact, the disorders can occur in combination with each other.

People with sound hypersensitivity disorders face many challenges when seeking professional help. Guidelines do not exist for clinical management of the disorders. Relatively few clinicians have training and experience in assessing and treating the disorders. Clinical management often requires the coordinated services of audiologists and psychological health providers. Most of all, professionals and the general public need resources with accurate and up-to-date information. This book and the references at the end of the book are resources that address these many challenges.

Notes to the Reader

This book is intended to provide educational information about sound hypersensitivity disorders, including loudness hyperacusis, pain hyperacusis, misophonia, noise sensitivity, and phonophobia. It cannot be construed as providing any form of therapy or treatment. If you have any of the symptoms described in this book and feel that professional services are needed, you should meet with an appropriate healthcare provider.

This book is referenced as for any scientific peer-reviewed article, with over 200 references cited. Professionals in the field of sound hypersensitivity disorders often disagree regarding many aspects of the disorders. The cited publications therefore express diverse opinions by the various authors. Any recommendations made for assessment, diagnosis, or treatment of sound hypersensitivity disorders should be considered in that light.

Artificial intelligence (AI) has not been used to write or edit any portion of this book, nor of any of the books in the Ears Gone Wrong® series.

PART 1

Introduction and Background

CHAPTER 1

Florence, Brian, and Lori

Florence

Florence is a 60-year-old mother of three and grandmother of two. Two of her boys were quite rambunctious growing up. One was diagnosed with a hyperactivity disorder, and Florence was continually trying to keep him calm and out of trouble. As a child, he would scream and yell loudly. Florence wore earplugs "to keep her ears from hurting." As the boys got older, they became interested in rock music. The one with hyperactivity was gifted a drum set, and his brother bought an electric guitar. Loud music became part of the daily household experience, and Florence continued to wear earplugs because of "all the racket."

Florence's children grew up and left home to pursue their own lives. She mostly stayed at home and "relished the quiet" she had missed for so many years. When she went out for a walk, or to drive her car, she realized everyday sounds seemed uncomfortably loud. She would routinely wear earplugs whenever she ventured outdoors to avoid the discomfort. She wore them so much that they interfered with her ability to communicate with her family and friends, which left her feeling isolated. Unbeknownst to her, she also had age-related hearing loss that contributed to her frustration.

At one point, Florence made an appointment with an audiologist to see if anything could be done that would allow her to hear her family and friends better and reduce her dependence on earplugs. The audiologist explained to her that wearing earplugs was depriving her ears of normal sound, which can create additional problems. That is, blocking sound with the earplugs made her ears *more* sensitive to sound, which only *worsened* her sound sensitivity problem. The audiologist asked if sound caused a sharp, jabbing pain. She said it didn't and explained that all sounds become uncomfortable for her when they reach a certain level. By "uncomfortable" she meant that when any sound reached a certain loudness level, it caused an overall feeling of discomfort in her head that she could not tolerate.

The audiologist conducted an extensive interview with Florence that focused on understanding her sound tolerance concerns. He also evaluated her hearing and determined that she had a mild hearing loss. He explained that she seemed to have *loudness hyperacusis* and not *pain hyperacusis*, which would have been implicated if she had sharp, jabbing pain. He also noted that her extensive use of earplugs suggested she might be experiencing *phonophobia* (unhealthy fear of sound).

The audiologist recommended treating the loudness hyperacusis by gradually reducing her use of earplugs and maintaining a constant environment of low-level, comfortable sound. He also suggested that she purchase a pair of custom-fit, high-fidelity (musician) earplugs, which would enable her to communicate better while still protecting her ears from sound that is uncomfortably loud.

The audiologist explained that complying with these suggestions would be a first step toward becoming more comfortable with normal levels of sound. He said that progress should be noted within a month or two. If progress was not evident within that period of time, then he might recommend using wearable sound generators or hearing aids with built-in sound generators. He was reluctant to recommend them right away because of their cost.

Florence followed the audiologist's suggestions. She made a point of not wearing the earplugs unless they were absolutely necessary. In the process, she discovered that she did not need them as much as she had thought. She realized that she had been wearing the earplugs to ensure that no sound would be so loud as to cause discomfort. She also switched to using custom-fit musician earplugs that were provided by the audiologist. She appreciated how the earplugs allowed her to communicate more easily with people when she was in louder environments. She could even go to restaurants and carry on a conversation around the table while wearing the earplugs.

At her appointment with the audiologist two months later, she was happy to report that her use of earplugs had been reduced by "at least 50 percent." Because of her progress, wearable devices were not recommended and she was advised to just continue her gradual reduction of earplug use. She met with the audiologist four months after that and reported that her earplug use was minimal and her loudness hyperacusis was not a significant problem anymore. She said, "I am no longer fearful of sound bothering me. I just carry my musician earplugs everywhere I go, and I know I will always have them if I need them."

Brian

Brian is a 55-year-old stockbroker. He has a family at home and goes into the office every day. He retired from the Army after being deployed on missions in Iraq and Afghanistan. His combat experiences were traumatic, and he suffered from post-traumatic stress disorder (PTSD). He received regular treatment for PTSD at his regional Veterans Affairs (VA) hospital.

The treatment Brian received for his PTSD was successful. He was able to sleep at night without being fearful. His panic attacks stopped, and he felt peaceful most of the time. One issue remained—he was sensitive to sound in general. Many sounds caused anxiety, especially sudden sounds like a door slamming, a dog barking, or someone honking at him while driving. He avoided any gathering of people because crowd noise caused him to be anxious.

As a result of these anxieties caused by sound, Brian returned to his VA psychologist. He told her that he only felt safe in quiet places. He drove to work every day and looked forward to spending the day in his quiet office. He would often stay late because he feared just walking to his car would expose him to sudden noises. At home, his family was fully aware that he was hypersensitive to sound, and they respectfully spoke in quiet voices and tried not to create any sudden sounds. Brian would watch TV at a very low volume with the closed-captioning turned on so that he could read the dialogue on screen. He rarely joined his family to go shopping, eat at restaurants, or even go on vacation.

The psychologist conducted an interview with Brian that focused on sound tolerance concerns. She determined that Brian's problem was one of *noise sensitivity* combined with *phonophobia* (excessive fear of sound). She understood that he did not react to any sound in particular, nor were his reactions dependent on the loudness of sound. Sound *in general* was annoying to him, and for that reason he lived his life mostly avoiding sound.

The psychologist's treatment was to add low-level comfortable sounds to his everyday environments—especially sounds that were interesting to him. He could listen to enjoyable music in the morning while getting ready for work. In the car he could listen to an audiobook or an interesting podcast. In his office she suggested adding a tabletop sound generator that could produce a variety of nature sounds (which would not distract him from his work). While at home she suggested gradually turning up the volume on the TV and listening carefully to what people were saying and not relying on the captioning. While lying in bed at night he could listen to an audiobook and also have sound from a tabletop sound generator running all night long.

The psychologist stressed to Brian that he should not try all of these things at once. He should try one thing at a time and only use sound that was comfortable to him. Little by little, he could add different sounds and also turn up the volume. She also recommended having a pair of custom-fit musician earplugs provided by an audiologist so that he could carry them in his pocket to be prepared for any situation that involved any sounds that are challenging.

Brian followed through with the psychologist's recommendations. It took some time, but he started to make notable progress. He kept reporting back to the psychologist, and she continued to provide suggestions to support his efforts. His reactions to sound became less and less, and he was able to live a more normal life and participate in activities with his family. To their delight, he was able to join them on a two-week vacation.

Lori

Lori is a 33-year-old schoolteacher. She has been teaching elementary school since she graduated from college. She grew up in a large family and had three sisters and two brothers. Family meals were a problem for her because the sounds of people eating caused her to feel anxious. She was especially annoyed by her brothers, who "purposely smacked their lips to get a reaction." Often, she would take her food and eat in her bedroom.

In college, she shared a dorm room for the first two years. It always made her anxious when her roommate ate in the room. Other sounds also became bothersome, such as pen clicking, foot tapping, and keyboard sounds. She would often go to the library where it was quiet. During her third year of college, she got her own apartment where she could control the environment. She would go to classes and then return to her apartment, where she ate all her meals.

Following college, Lori got a job teaching fourth grade. She brought her own lunch every day and usually ate it in her classroom when the children were in the cafeteria. She avoided the teachers' break room because her colleagues usually snacked and drank coffee in there. This has been her situation for the past 10 years.

She finally decided to seek professional help. She started by making an appointment with a psychologist. The psychologist did not know anything about her condition but was willing to learn. Lori shared what she had learned on the internet. She suspected she had *misophonia*, which would explain why she reacted to eating and other human-made sounds. The psychologist knew of an audiologist who specialized in treating tinnitus and hyperacusis, and thought he might be able to help. Lori met with the audiologist, who confirmed her condition was indeed misophonia. He started her on a program of sound therapy, and she continued to meet with the psychologist, who provided cognitive behavioral therapy (CBT). Over time her condition improved, and she was able to tolerate the sounds that had been so bothersome for most of her life.

Where Do We Go from Here?

This book covers five distinctly different sound hypersensitivity disorders: loudness hyperacusis, pain hyperacusis, misophonia, noise sensitivity, and phonophobia. The three "case studies" (Florence, Brian, and Lori) exemplify all of these disorders except for pain hyperacusis (which was ruled out in Florence's case).

Each of the case studies had successful outcomes. The treatment they received was beneficial to them, and their lives were significantly improved as a result. These are of course ideal scenarios that may not reflect reality for some people suffering from sound hypersensitivity disorders. It's not that these people can't be helped—the challenge is finding a clinician who truly understands the disorders, how they differ, and how to provide effective clinical services. Readers of this book may end up knowing more about sound hypersensitivity disorders than many professionals in the field. That is certainly not a bad thing because awareness of the facts is key to making informed decisions.

It can be difficult to find "the facts" pertaining to sound hypersensitivity disorders, especially when relying on the internet for information. The best source of facts—although far from perfect—is the relevant peer-reviewed literature that contains articles written by scientists, critiqued by their peers, and published in scientific journals. In this book I refer often to the literature as well as to what I have learned during my 35-year career as an auditory researcher. My approach is to present facts along with opinions based on the facts. I rely largely on PubMed to obtain pertinent information.

PubMed is an "online database with abstracts of medical articles, hosted by US National Library of Medicine" (pubmed.ncbi.nlm.nih.gov). Searching for articles on PubMed identifies peer-reviewed publications that pertain to the topic of interest. These publications represent the "scientific literature." To write this book I have continually searched for articles on PubMed for the most scientifically based information that's available to date. The book is written with the same rigor I've always used to write scientific articles during my research career. The only difference is, I have tried to make the book understandable by anyone—professionals and the lay public alike.

Suggestions for Getting the Most Benefit from This Book

If you have, or suspect you have, a problem tolerating sound, then you might want to first focus on chapter 2, which compares and contrasts the different sound hypersensitivity disorders. You may relate to one of these disorders more than the others. If so, then you can turn to the chapters that address that particular disorder.

Other readers may include clinicians, researchers, college professors, and anyone who just wants to understand these different sound hypersensitivity disorders and what options are available for their clinical management. Chapter 2 provides a high-level overview of the different disorders. Chapter 3 describes common misconceptions relating to their clinical assessment. Chapter 4 mentions several overarching concerns when diagnosing any sound hypersensitivity disorder. In chapter 5, the assessment process is described in detail. Whereas many questionnaires have been developed, it is argued that the best information to understand a person's unique condition comes from a targeted, in-depth interview. The Sound Hypersensitivity Interview is suggested for this purpose. In chapter 5, each question from the Sound Hypersensitivity Interview is described along with how different responses might indicate which sound hypersensitivity disorder(s) is experienced.

Following chapter 5, the focus shifts to *diagnosing* each of the disorders: loudness hyperacusis (chapter 6), pain hyperacusis (chapter 7), misophonia (chapter 8), noise sensitivity (chapter 9), and phonophobia (chapter 10).

The subsequent section focuses on treatment. Chapter 11 discusses considerations relating to treatment in general. Starting with chapter 12, treatment of the five sound hypersensitivity disorders is described—each in its own chapter: loudness hyperacusis (chapter 12), pain hyperacusis (chapter 13), misophonia (chapter 14), noise sensitivity (chapter 15), and phonophobia (chapter 16). Chapter 17 provides a brief overall summary along with suggestions and resources.

The Big Picture

The primary area of focus during my career was clinical assessment and treatment of tinnitus. That field has made great strides over the past 50 years, but we still don't have clinical standards nor any system for certifying clinicians for competency. The concerns about tinnitus not having standards nor a certification system are even greater for sound hypersensitivity disorders. The disorders are inconsistently labeled and defined. Some professionals consider all of the different disorders to be "hyperacusis," and they are treated as one and the same disorder. Others stick with the term *hyperacusis* but describe different types of hyperacusis.[1,2]

We are fortunately seeing a great deal of interest in sound hypersensitivity disorders. Many articles have been published and, increasingly, more books are dedicated to the topic. Tinnitus conferences and meetings generally include sections and talks specific to sound hypersensitivity disorders. Organizations also exist to promote relevant education and research.

For now, we need to rely on what has been researched and written about sound hypersensitivity disorders along with the opinions of credible professionals in the field. My hope is that this book will bring some clarity about what is known and ultimately help those who are unable to tolerate everyday sounds that saturate our environment.

CHAPTER 2

Sound Hypersensitivity Disorders—An Overview

In the conclusion to chapter 1, it is pointed out that the field of sound hypersensitivity disorders is in an early stage of development. The scientific literature does not use consistent terms and definitions to describe these disorders. There is not even agreement as to how to refer to the field in general. For example, it is referred to as:

- sound tolerance conditions/disorders
- decreased/lowered/poor sound tolerance
- sound/auditory intolerance
- sound sensitivity
- hypersensitivity to sound
- auditory hypersensitivity disorders, etc.

The word most often used is *hyperacusis*, which has various meanings and often is used as an umbrella term to include all sound hypersensitivity disorders. This inconsistency in terminology and definitions poses significant challenges to anyone seeking help. Clinicians who provide services for these disorders vary greatly with respect to how they go about assessment, diagnosis, and treatment.[3]

My experience over the years as an auditory researcher and my awareness of the scientific literature have led me to conclude that there are five sound hypersensitivity disorders. Two of them (loudness hyperacusis and pain hyperacusis) involve hypersensitivity to the loudness of sound, meaning that sounds are uncomfortably or painfully loud that are otherwise fine for most people. Two of the disorders (misophonia and noise sensitivity) involve emotional reactions to sound, meaning that certain sounds trigger emotional responses such as annoyance or anger. The fifth (phonophobia) is the state of excessive and persistent fear that sound will *cause* discomfort and/or emotional reactions. We will briefly summarize each of these disorders in this chapter. Later chapters will describe the different disorders in greater detail.

Loudness Hyperacusis

Loudness hyperacusis is physical discomfort that results from exposure to any sound that reaches a certain intensity level that would be comfortably tolerated by the average person.[4] It's necessary to distinguish loudness hyperacusis from pain hyperacusis.[3] With loudness hyperacusis, the physical discomfort is localized to the head as an unbearable sensation. Pain hyperacusis has been described as "a burning, stabbing, jabbing pain that feels like someone is pushing hot pokers into their ears."[5]

Loudness hyperacusis is the most common form of hyperacusis. It is characterized by an inability to tolerate sounds at low to moderate intensity levels—sounds that are easily tolerated by most people. Treatment is usually straightforward and involves gradual exposure to increasing levels of sound. Patients may be fit with ear-level sound generators or hearing aids with built-in sound generators. The systematic use of sound can usually increase a person's ability to tolerate sounds at greater intensity levels over time.

Pain Hyperacusis

Pain hyperacusis is a more severe form of hyperacusis and in fact is a "completely different subcategory."[5] "[L]oudness passes some threshold and turns into actual pain. And that pain lingers and worsens. It's impossible to describe how much suffering this condition entails."[6] Pain hyperacusis is especially challenging to the sufferer and is often misunderstood by the professional community.

To briefly explain what might cause the pain (more on this later), the inner ear (cochlea) is connected to the brain stem by the auditory nerve. This nerve is a bundle of nerve fibers, some of which have characteristics that would make them function like pain receptors.[7] These fibers may be the source of the pain, but there are other possible sources.

Importantly, people with pain hyperacusis may not do well with sound therapy, which would be the treatment of choice for loudness hyperacusis.[5] However, studies have not yet evaluated sound therapy (or earplug use) for pain hyperacusis. It may be that sound therapy is less effective for these patients based on preliminary studies, but we do not yet have definitive evidence. Pain hyperacusis is a very complex disorder that is more fully described in chapter 7.

Misophonia

Both forms of hyperacusis involve hypersensitivity to the loudness of sound. Misophonia is hypersensitivity to *specific sounds, regardless of their loudness.*[8] Misophonia is characterized by certain sounds causing intense feelings of annoyance, anger, disgust, etc.[9] The sounds may also cause physical responses such as tightened muscles, racing heart, and difficulty breathing.[10] Most typically, sounds that trigger the reactions come from the human body, such as sounds made by people eating. Other sounds could include foot tapping, repeated pen clicking, and typing.

It needs to be emphasized that *misophonia has nothing to do with the loudness of sounds.* Sounds that trigger the reactions are psychologically upsetting. Many factors may influence the response, such as previous experiences relating to the sound, the subjective meaning of the sound, and the context in which the sound appears.[10] It can be a complex problem requiring both audiology and psychology intervention.

Noise Sensitivity

Like misophonia, noise sensitivity is not a problem tolerating the loudness of sound. It has been described as the physiological and psychological state of a person that increases reactivity to noise *in general*.[11] "In general" distinguishes noise sensitivity from misophonia, which is characterized by emotional reactions to *specific* sounds.

Compared to the general public, noise-sensitive people are more likely to be annoyed by noise, awakened by noise, and to pay more attention to sounds in general.[11] As a consequence, they have greater difficulty habituating to (learning to ignore) sounds in the environment that have no relevance for performing daily activities. Noise sensitivity is commonly seen in people who have psychological disorders such as anxiety, depression, autism spectrum disorder, and traumatic brain injury.

Phonophobia

Phonophobia does not pertain to adverse *reactions* to sound but rather to a state of *fear* that sound will cause discomfort, distress, or pain.[12] Phonophobia is difficult to define because *phobia* refers to *unhealthy* fear.[13-15] People with any of the above four sound hypersensitivity disorders may have a *healthy* concern that sound will be uncomfortable. For example, a person with severe hyperacusis might wear earplugs when walking next to a busy street because of the likelihood of sudden loud sounds. The healthy concern becomes unhealthy fear when the person is so fearful as to constantly avoid sound even when there's no chance of being exposed to uncomfortable sound.

It is sensible to protect against sound in an environment that is likely to have sounds that are uncomfortably loud or that cause negative emotional reactions. This becomes an important issue when treating a person for a sound hypersensitivity disorder. The person needs to know how to go about protecting against uncomfortable sound but not *overprotecting,* which would mean avoiding sound or wearing hearing protection unnecessarily. We will have much more to say about this in the upcoming chapters.

Summary

These brief descriptions of the five sound hypersensitivity disorders may have left the reader with more questions than answers. That would be understandable because the differences between the disorders can be subtle, and terminology and definitions vary so much. As already pointed out, the scientific literature is relied upon for most of the information presented in this book. Otherwise, ideas and concepts are tied together in a manner that makes the most sense given the inconsistency in the field.

The main thing to remember is that sound hypersensitivity disorders really are uniquely distinguishable and it is inappropriate to refer to them all as "hyperacusis." Most generally, the loudness of sound can be a problem if sounds are perceived as unbearably loud when they seem normal to other people. That would describe loudness hyperacusis.

Pain hyperacusis is similar except sound causes piercing pain in the ear. Distinguishing between loudness hyperacusis and pain hyperacusis is critical because they require very different approaches to treatment.

The loudness of sound is irrelevant when the sound hypersensitivity disorder is characterized mainly by negative emotional reactions to the sound. These disorders are misophonia and noise sensitivity. Misophonia involves emotional reactions to specific sounds while noise sensitivity means the person is bothered by sound in general. Treatment is similar for these two conditions.

Phonophobia is a separate category from the other four sound hypersensitivity disorders, and yet it can co-exist with any of them. We distinguished between a healthy concern for sound being uncomfortable and an unhealthy fear of sound that can be incapacitating.

In the next section (part 2) we will focus on assessment of people who complain of sound hypersensitivity. Many different questionnaires have been developed, and they will be mentioned and briefly described. The most important concern when conducting the assessment is understanding how sound actually affects the person in daily life. That will be the focus in chapter 5.

PART 2

Assessment of Sound Hypersensitivity

CHAPTER 3

Common Misconceptions

Assessment procedures are necessary to determine whether a person has one or more sound hypersensitivity disorders and whether treatment is necessary. These next three chapters address various aspects that are relevant to assessing anyone complaining of hypersensitivity to sound.

The present chapter describes common misconceptions that can compromise the assessment and lead to an inaccurate diagnosis. Chapter 4 explains important considerations that pertain to the assessment process. Chapter 5 describes specific approaches that can be used to screen for a sound hypersensitivity disorder and to perform a comprehensive assessment.

The following concerns are common misconceptions to be aware of prior to an assessment being done.

1. Any complaint of sound hypersensitivity should be taken seriously. Depending on the circumstances, however, some complaints do not meet the definition of a sound hypersensitivity *disorder*.

2. A common measure of sound sensitivity is loudness discomfort level (LDL) testing. Although this testing is often performed by audiologists, it is not reliable for assessing real-life hypersensitivity to sound.

3. Questionnaires have been developed to assess sound hypersensitivity disorders. These questionnaires have value for assessing specific disorders but are inadequate for distinguishing between the different disorders.

4. A *consensus definition of hyperacusis* was published.[16] Whereas that definition works well for sound hypersensitivity in general, it is not specific to hyperacusis.

These four common misconceptions are explained below. Further details about misconceptions #2 and #3 are provided in appendixes A and B, respectively.

When Sound Hypersensitivity Is Not a "Disorder"

Hypothetically, everyone can be placed somewhere on a sound sensitivity scale—from "I'm never annoyed by any sound" to "Almost every sound causes discomfort." At what point on this scale does common annoyance become a sound hypersensitivity *disorder*? This question is not easily answered, but some examples can be helpful.

Common Annoyance from Everyday Sounds

Most people are annoyed by *some* sounds—like a squeaky rocking chair, a constant rattle while driving, and a dripping water faucet. We can usually take action to reduce or eliminate such mildly irritating sounds. Some people are annoyed by sounds they cannot avoid—like leaf blowers, babies crying, and traffic noise. We all live with sounds we prefer not to hear. The next seven chapters focus on how to determine whether a person actually has a sound hypersensitivity disorder and not just common annoyance from everyday sounds.

Hearing Aids

People who wear hearing aids (especially new users) often complain that the hearing aids are "too loud." Such a complaint is usually an indication that the hearing aids need to be adjusted so that all amplified sounds are in a comfortable range.[17] This is something audiologists can take care of. In some cases, however, amplified sound is not well tolerated and may be an indication the person has loudness hyperacusis.[18]

Loudness Recruitment

Loudness recruitment is a technical term that is explained in appendix C. The term needs to be mentioned because it has been used incorrectly as meaning the same thing as loudness hyperacusis. Loudness recruitment is not a sound hypersensitivity disorder.[9] To understand loudness recruitment, it is important to understand the concept of *dynamic range,* which is the range of decibels between the threshold of hearing sensitivity and the level at which sound becomes uncomfortably loud. Please see appendix C for an explanation of dynamic range and how it relates to loudness recruitment.

Loudness Discomfort Level (LDL) Testing

Loudness discomfort levels (LDLs) are often measured by audiologists to evaluate people with suspected loudness hyperacusis.[19] The testing involves raising the level of a tone or a band of noise in small steps and asking the person to report when the sound is uncomfortably loud (or *about to become* uncomfortably loud). (Appendix A provides more detail about LDL testing.) For a number of reasons, LDL testing is not normally recommended for this purpose.[4] Perhaps most importantly, studies have shown that LDLs do not necessarily predict a sound hypersensitivity disorder.[20-22] Another concern is that any coexisting tinnitus (which is likely) might be made worse as a result of the testing.[4] Further, people with a complaint of sound hypersensitivity who are tested for LDLs are those who would be least likely to be comfortable with such testing.[19] Because of these concerns it is difficult to justify testing routinely for LDLs.

Sound Hypersensitivity Questionnaires

This is a topic that requires listing and summarizing the questionnaires that are available to measure the different sound hypersensitivity disorders. There are so many that is not possible to review them in this chapter. They cannot be left out, however, so this information is provided in appendix B for the interested reader.

Appendix B covers many of the questionnaires that have been validated for assessing sound hypersensitivity disorders. In the appendix, eight questionnaires address hyperacusis, six address misophonia, two address noise sensitivity, and two address phonophobia. The hyperacusis questionnaires do not distinguish between loudness hyperacusis and pain hyperacusis—at least with respect to how these disorders are described in this book.

No questionnaire is available that is capable of determining which sound hypersensitivity disorder, or combination of disorders, may be experienced by an individual. Only a comprehensive interview can provide the information necessary to distinguish between the different disorders and identify which are likely to explain a person's symptoms. In chapter 5 the Sound Hypersensitivity Interview is described question-by-question as well as how responses to each question might contribute to diagnosing any of the five sound hypersensitivity disorders.

Consensus Definition of Hyperacusis

A study was conducted because "There is currently no singularly accepted definition of hyperacusis."[16] (p. 607) To obtain consensus, the investigators used the *Delphi method*, which is a scientific method of obtaining opinions and feedback from experts regarding a particular issue.[23] They agreed on a definition of hyperacusis: *"A reduced tolerance to sound(s) that are perceived as normal to the majority of the population or were perceived as normal to the person before their onset of hyperacusis, where 'normal' refers to sounds that are generally well tolerated."* (p. 610)

A close examination of this consensus definition reveals that it could apply as an overarching definition for loudness hyperacusis, pain hyperacusis, misophonia, and noise sensitivity—disorders that can all be thought of as "reduced tolerance to sound." The definition would not apply to phonophobia because phonophobia is not a reaction to sound but rather *fear* of sound.

The investigators acknowledged that misophonia and phonophobia are "separate conditions to hyperacusis."[16] Their consensus statement may be helpful in providing a broad definition of sound hypersensitivity disorders, but it does not distinguish between the different disorders.

Summary

Guidelines do not exist to assess and diagnose sound hypersensitivity disorders. Clinicians may rely on specialized questionnaires for this purpose. Most of the questionnaires that are currently available are summarized in appendix B. Some are appropriate for testing for specific disorders, but none can differentiate between the disorders. It is recommended to use the Sound Hypersensitivity Interview (chapter 5), which focuses on determining how sound hypersensitivity affects a person's daily activities. With a clear understanding of how the disorders differ, the Interview helps to make an accurate diagnosis.

CHAPTER 4

Making the Diagnosis: Important Considerations

As mentioned in the last chapter, it is common for people to complain of certain sounds being annoying or irritating. At what point does annoyance or other emotional reactions to sound indicate the person has misophonia or noise sensitivity? Some people just don't like noisy environments. Do they have noise sensitivity? Loudness hyperacusis? How do we distinguish between common, everyday dislike for certain sounds (or sound in general) and an actual sound hypersensitivity *disorder*? One research group stated that the goal is to define "discrete subtypes that can be unambiguously differentiated."[24]

THE HYPERACUSIS AND MISOPHONIA BOOK

Working Definition of a Sound Hypersensitivity Disorder

Let's start with a working definition of a sound hypersensitivity disorder that would apply to each and all of the individual disorders: *A sound hypersensitivity disorder is defined by interference with, or prevention of, participation in normal life activities because everyday sounds cause physical discomfort, pain, negative emotional reactions, excessive fear, or some combination of these symptoms.*

In chapters 6 through 10, working definitions for each of the five sound hypersensitivity disorders are provided. They are referred to as *working definitions* because they work for our purposes and are not necessarily definitions that would be used by others. The use of working definitions is unavoidable because terminology and definitions for sound hypersensitivity disorders are so variable between clinics and researchers.

Medical Conditions That Can Be Associated with Sound Hypersensitivity Disorders

Many medical conditions can be associated with sound hypersensitivity disorders. Clinicians should be aware if any of these conditions co-occur with a sound hypersensitivity disorder and determine if they are linked in some way.

How many causes of sound hypersensitivity disorders are there? We do not know the answer to that question, and the list of *possible* causes is extensive. One author has created a list of medical conditions that have "a suggested association with hyperacusis."[25] That list contains 16 disease classifications, which include 60 specific diseases or conditions that have been reported to be linked with "disorders of sound tolerance."

Trying to understand the *cause* of a person's sound hypersensitivity disorder will often be a futile effort. It can be productive, however, to determine the person's coexisting (comorbid) conditions that might be linked to the disorder. Some of the more relevant conditions are described in appendix E. Treatment of any sound hypersensitivity disorder should address the specific disorder along with any associated medical conditions.

Identifying the Primary Disorder to Prioritize Treatment

People with a sound hypersensitivity disorder cannot live a normal life due to *physical discomfort* (including pain) and/or *emotional reactions* (usually anxiety but also any other negative emotions). The physical discomfort is due to loudness hyperacusis or pain hyperacusis. The emotional reactions are due to any of the disorders but are the primary problem with misophonia, noise sensitivity, and phonophobia. An accurate diagnosis is essential to determine which method of treatment would be most appropriate. It is therefore essential to identify the primary disorder. Any secondary disorders also need to be identified.

The following three generalizations are important to keep in mind.

1. If the person is diagnosed with loudness hyperacusis or pain hyperacusis, the physical discomfort would likely lead to negative emotions such as frustration, anxiety, and fear. *The physical discomfort is the primary disorder.* Any associated negative emotions might be serious enough to be considered a secondary disorder. It might be natural to think that a person with loudness hyperacusis who "dislikes sound" also has misophonia. Using the working definitions in this book, it would be unusual for a person with loudness hyperacusis to also have misophonia.

2. If the person is diagnosed with misophonia or noise sensitivity, the emotional reactions are not likely to lead to physical discomfort. It would therefore be unusual for the person to also have loudness hyperacusis or pain hyperacusis. *The emotional reactions are the primary disorder.* Physical discomfort would not normally be a concern.

3. If the person is diagnosed with phonophobia, the root cause of the excessive fear needs to be determined. The root cause will likely be one or more of the other sound hypersensitivity disorders—loudness hyperacusis, pain hyperacusis, misophonia, and/or noise sensitivity. *The primary disorder is whichever of the five sound hypersensitivity disorders has the greatest impact on the person's life.* Any coexisting disorders would be considered secondary.

Degree of Life Impact

If a person has been evaluated using the Sound Hypersensitivity Interview (chapter 5), and our working definition of one of the disorders accurately describes the person's symptoms, then that person can be reasonably diagnosed as having that particular disorder. The next question is the *degree* to which the disorder impacts the person's life. We can use the following definitions as a rough guide to diagnose a mild, moderate, severe, or extreme sound hypersensitivity disorder:

- *Mild disorder* = minimal but significant interference with normal life activities.
- *Moderate disorder* = substantial interference with normal life activities.
- *Severe disorder* = extensive interference with normal life activities.
- *Extreme disorder* = prevents most or all normal life activities.

The exact wording of these definitions is less important than the clinician's judgment as to the existence of the disorder and the degree to which the disorder impacts the person's life. The objective of conducting the assessment and making the diagnosis is to assist in determining what would be the best approach to restore the person's quality of life to what it was prior to experiencing the symptoms. The person's quality of life is what ultimately matters.

Borderline Cases

It can be difficult to diagnose a healthcare condition when the symptoms exist at a very low level. For example, many people experience pain on a regular basis, which may or may not be considered a *chronic pain disorder* requiring treatment. As another example, tinnitus has been defined as "ear noise lasting at least five minutes and occurring at least weekly."[26] Sounds in the ears or head that do not meet this definition are considered *ear noise*. Tinnitus is a medical condition warranting clinical services. Ear noise is not a medical condition.

Turning back to sound hypersensitivity, a number of questions speak to the difficulty of diagnosing an actual *disorder*. When does being *bothered by sound* become a healthcare disorder that warrants being assessed and possibly treated? More specifically, what are the symptoms that would be necessary to diagnose:

- being bothered by the loudness of sound as *loudness hyperacusis*?
- having pain in the ears as *pain hyperacusis*?
- being bothered by specific sounds as *misophonia*?
- being overwhelmed by sound in general as *noise sensitivity*?
- avoiding sound as *phonophobia*?

These questions do not have clear answers, which is what the next chapters in the next section (part 3) intend to address. The professional field of sound hypersensitivity disorders is too early in its growth to have established terminology, definitions, and criteria for making diagnoses. We must therefore rely on working definitions. Chapters 6 through 10 each focus on how to diagnose one of the five sound hypersensitivity disorders. Working definitions for these disorders are provided at the beginning of each chapter. If a person has symptoms meeting one of the definitions, then diagnosing the particular disorder would be appropriate. It is of course not that simple—the clinician must be knowledgeable about all of the disorders, how they differ, and how to conduct the assessment to make an accurate diagnosis.

The Sound Hypersensitivity Interview is a recommended tool to capture the relevant information to determine whether a person has a sound hypersensitivity disorder. The Interview is described question-by-question in the next chapter. In most cases, conducting the Interview will answer the questions asked above—*what are the symptoms that would be necessary to diagnose a sound hypersensitivity disorder?*

We started this chapter with a working definition of sound hypersensitivity disorders in general: *A sound hypersensitivity disorder is defined by interference with, or prevention of, participation in normal life activities because everyday sounds cause physical discomfort, negative emotional reactions, excessive fear, or some combination of these symptoms.* This definition would not apply to *borderline cases* who are bothered by, or fearful of, sound but not to the degree as to interfere significantly with normal life activities. It is therefore essential to conduct the in-depth Interview to fully understand how a person's complaints actually relate to the person's life activities. At the end of the Interview, the person should be asked, "Do you feel that treatment for your sound hypersensitivity would be helpful?" If so, then treatment should be made available.

CHAPTER 5

The Sound Hypersensitivity Interview

The Sound Hypersensitivity Interview is a rather lengthy interview that may require up to an hour to complete. It is intended to be administered face-to-face for maximum effectiveness. It should not normally be self-administered because of the difficulty a person might have interpreting the responses. It can, however, be completed by an individual and then sent to a clinician for interpretation and diagnosis purposes—which would probably still require a conversation to clarify the responses.

This chapter lists each question along with a description of the question's intent, possible response choices, and how to interpret the different responses. Each question adds insight to a person's possible sound hypersensitivity disorder. The combination of questions should be adequate to make a diagnosis of loudness hyperacusis, pain hyperacusis, misophonia, noise sensitivity, and/or phonophobia.

This of course assumes the person has undergone a full evaluation by an audiologist.

There are actually two levels of assessment for sound hypersensitivity. Screening, which is the lowest level, is done to determine whether it seems likely, or even possible, that a person has a sound hypersensitivity disorder. If so, then a comprehensive assessment is necessary to make a diagnosis or to rule out all of the potential disorders.

Screening for a Sound Hypersensitivity Disorder

In each of my first three books in the Ears Gone Wrong® series, I provide a detailed explanation of the Tinnitus and Hearing Survey.[26-28] I always suggest using the Tinnitus and Hearing Survey because it is so effective and efficient in identifying how people perceive their own auditory problems. This one-page survey normally takes just a couple of minutes to complete. Its main purpose is to determine whether a person has a significant problem with tinnitus that is not being blamed on hearing difficulties.[29]

An additional purpose is to screen for a sound hypersensitivity disorder. The person is asked if sounds are too loud or uncomfortable when they seem normal to others. If this is at least a "small problem" (that is not due to hearing aids), then the person is asked to list two examples of these kinds of sounds. If a real problem is suggested by the person's responses, then a full evaluation can be completed using the Sound Hypersensitivity Interview.[4] (The Tinnitus and Hearing Survey is available as a free download on the Resources page at https://www.earsgonewrong.org/)

Sound Tolerance Interview

The Sound Hypersensitivity Interview is an adaptation of the Sound Tolerance Interview, which was originally published in the clinician's handbook for Progressive Tinnitus Management.[30] The Sound Tolerance Interview was developed specifically for assessing hyperacusis and was revised to also assess for misophonia, noise sensitivity, and phonophobia.[4] I have further revised it and renamed it the Sound Hypersensitivity Interview.

Sound Hypersensitivity Interview: Question by Question

The Sound Hypersensitivity Interview should be used only if a person has made a credible complaint of sound hypersensitivity. Ideally, the person would have been screened for sound hypersensitivity using the Tinnitus and Hearing Survey—as described above. The Interview is used to evaluate the person's symptoms and determine if they reflect one or more of the sound hypersensitivity disorders. It can also be used following treatment to evaluate for changes in the symptoms.

The Interview contains nine questions. Some of the questions are straightforward and others require detailed answers. We will now go through each question as shown on the Interview form, discuss the possible answers, and explain how each answer might suggest the person experiences one or more sound hypersensitivity disorders. (The Sound Hypersensitivity Interview is available as a free download on the Resources page at https://www.ears-gonewrong.org/)

1. Do you wear hearing aids?	
☐ No – go to Question 2	☐ Yes
(If YES) Are everyday sounds too loud when you are wearing your hearing aids?	
☐ No	☐ Yes
(If YES) Are everyday sounds too loud when you are not wearing your hearing aids?	
☐ No	☐ Yes

Question 1 is only relevant if the person wears hearing aids. If so, the purpose is to determine whether everyday sounds are too loud when wearing the hearing aids. If they are, then the follow-up question asks if everyday sounds are too loud when *not* wearing the hearing aids. If the complaint is specific to amplified sound and otherwise is not a concern, that would usually indicate that the hearing aids need to be adjusted so that all amplified sounds are in a comfortable range (as mentioned in chapter 3).[17] It also would suggest that loudness hyperacusis is not experienced by that person. In some cases, however, amplified sound is not well tolerated and may be an indication that the person has loudness hyperacusis.[18]

2. Is there anything you *want* to be doing, but *are not* doing because of difficulty tolerating sound?

This is an *open-ended* question, meaning there are no response options to choose from. Open-ended questions can quickly identify a person's most significant concern. This question is therefore asked before any examples are provided of how sound hypersensitivity can affect life activities.

3. Have you used any of the following to help with difficulty tolerating sound? If so, please indicate *how helpful* **on a scale of 0 to 10.** *("0" = not at all; "10" = extremely helpful)*

☐ Using background sound

How helpful?	0	1	2	3	4	5	6	7	8	9	10

☐ Gradually listening to the types of sounds that are uncomfortable to get used to them

How helpful?	0	1	2	3	4	5	6	7	8	9	10

☐ Relaxation techniques

How helpful?	0	1	2	3	4	5	6	7	8	9	10

☐ Medications

How helpful?	0	1	2	3	4	5	6	7	8	9	10

☐ Counseling

How helpful?	0	1	2	3	4	5	6	7	8	9	10

☐ Lifestyle changes to create quieter environments

How helpful?	0	1	2	3	4	5	6	7	8	9	10

☐ Other_____

How helpful?	0	1	2	3	4	5	6	7	8	9	10

If properly screened, the person responding to the interview questions most likely has a genuine sound hypersensitivity problem. Question 3 contains a list of possible approaches that might have been used in an attempt to lessen the problem. The helpfulness of any approach used is rated on a scale of 0 (*not at all helpful*) to 10 (*extremely helpful*). If the person is diagnosed with a sound hypersensitivity disorder, this information will be helpful for tailoring a treatment program that takes into account any treatments that have been tried.

4. How much does difficulty tolerating sound affect your life? *("0" = not at all; "10" = as much as you can imagine)*

0	1	2	3	4	5	6	7	8	9	10

Question 4 provides an overall rating of how much sound hypersensitivity impacts the person's life. This may be the key question to know how serious the problem is to the person. Does the person consider it a *slight* problem? A *mild* problem? A *moderate* problem? A *severe* problem? When we get to the chapters that describe treatment for sound hypersensitivity disorders, we'll talk about how treatment differs according to how much the disorder impacts the person's life. Anything up to a moderate problem may just require some counseling and lifestyle changes. In fact, a *slight* or a *mild* sound hypersensitivity problem may not even be diagnosed as a sound hypersensitivity *disorder*. A severe sound hypersensitivity disorder would generally require targeted treatment.

---

5. What kinds of sounds are bothersome to you? Why are they bothersome?

[Check all categories that apply; circle any sounds identified as a problem; write in any additional sounds that are not listed; for each category selected, select one or more of the reasons why the sound is uncomfortable.]

☐ High-pitched sounds (squeals, squeaks, beeps, whistles, rings, _____)
 ☐ too loud; ☐ painful; ☐ annoying; ☐ make me angry; ☐ make me anxious; ☐ overwhelming; ☐ I avoid
 Comments: _____

☐ Low-pitched sounds (bass from radio, next door music, _____)
 ☐ too loud; ☐ painful; ☐ annoying; ☐ make me angry; ☐ make me anxious; ☐ overwhelming; ☐ I avoid
 Comments: _____

☐ Traffic (warning) sounds (emergency vehicle sirens, car horns, back-up beeper on truck/van, _____)
 ☐ too loud; ☐ painful; ☐ annoying; ☐ make me angry; ☐ make me anxious; ☐ overwhelming; ☐ I avoid
 Comments: _____

☐ Traffic (background) sounds (road noise, road construction, diesel engines, garbage trucks, _____)
 ☐ too loud; ☐ painful; ☐ annoying; ☐ make me angry; ☐ make me anxious; ☐ overwhelming; ☐ I avoid
 Comments: _____

☐ Other background sounds (crowd noise, restaurant, city noise, sporting events, _____)
 ☐ too loud; ☐ painful; ☐ annoying; ☐ make me angry; ☐ make me anxious; ☐ overwhelming; ☐ I avoid
 Comments: _____

☐ Sudden-impact sounds (door slam, car backfiring, objects dropping on floor, dishes clattering, ____)
 ☐ too loud; ☐ painful; ☐ annoying; ☐ make me angry; ☐ make me anxious; ☐ overwhelming; ☐ I avoid
 Comments: _____

☐ Voices (television, radio, movies, children's voices, men's voices, women's voices, babies crying, __)
 ☐ too loud; ☐ painful; ☐ annoying; ☐ make me angry; ☐ make me anxious; ☐ overwhelming; ☐ I avoid
 Comments: _____

☐ Oral (mouth) sounds (chewing, breathing, swallowing, coughing, _____)
 ☐ too loud; ☐ painful; ☐ annoying; ☐ make me angry; ☐ make me anxious; ☐ overwhelming; ☐ I avoid
 Comments: _____

☐ Nasal (nose) sounds (sniffing, sniffling, breathing, snorting, _____)
 ☐ too loud; ☐ painful; ☐ annoying; ☐ make me angry; ☐ make me anxious; ☐ overwhelming; ☐ I avoid
 Comments: _____

☐ Human-movement sounds (pen clicking, wrappers crinkling, typing, foot tapping, finger snapping, ___)
 ☐ too loud; ☐ painful; ☐ annoying; ☐ make me angry; ☐ make me anxious; ☐ overwhelming; ☐ I avoid
 Comments: _____

☐ Other: _____
 ☐ too loud; ☐ painful; ☐ annoying; ☐ make me angry; ☐ make me anxious; ☐ overwhelming; ☐ I avoid
 Comments: _____

Question 5 contains a list of 10 different categories of sounds (plus *other*) that might be bothersome to the person. For each category, examples are given. Any example sound that is bothersome is circled, and any bothersome sound that is not listed is written in. Each category of sound also includes a list of possible reasons why those sounds are bothersome (*too loud, painful, annoying, make me angry, make me anxious, overwhelming, I avoid*). For any categories chosen, comments should be provided to further explain.

Responses to this series of questions are especially useful for differentiating between the five sound hypersensitivity disorders. The item drills down to the details of what general categories of sounds are bothersome, what specific sounds are bothersome within each category, and the reasons such sounds are bothersome. For example, if *too loud* is chosen for sounds that are not considered too loud by most people, then loudness hyperacusis is suspected. If sounds are *painful*, then it is important to define pain—if the pain is the "burning, stabbing, jabbing" type, then pain hyperacusis would be suspected. If oral, nasal, or human-movement sounds *make me angry*, misophonia would be suspected. If *other background sounds* such as crowd noise and restaurants are *overwhelming*, then noise sensitivity would be suspected. If the person checks *I avoid* in many instances, then phonophobia would be suspected. These examples of course are an oversimplification, but they show how the responses can be helpful in making the diagnosis.

6. During each of these activities, how often is difficulty tolerating sound a problem?

(Check "avoid" if the activity is avoided due to difficulty tolerating sound; if an activity is avoided, two boxes can be checked for that activity)

	Never	Rarely	Sometimes	Often	Always	N/A	Avoid
Concerts	☐	☐	☐	☐	☐	☐	☐
Watching movies in a theater	☐	☐	☐	☐	☐	☐	☐
Watching TV or movies at home	☐	☐	☐	☐	☐	☐	☐
Shopping	☐	☐	☐	☐	☐	☐	☐
Going to restaurants	☐	☐	☐	☐	☐	☐	☐
Attending religious services	☐	☐	☐	☐	☐	☐	☐
Work responsibilities	☐	☐	☐	☐	☐	☐	☐
Day-to-day responsibilities outside of work	☐	☐	☐	☐	☐	☐	☐
Driving	☐	☐	☐	☐	☐	☐	☐
Housekeeping activities	☐	☐	☐	☐	☐	☐	☐
Childcare	☐	☐	☐	☐	☐	☐	☐
Social activities	☐	☐	☐	☐	☐	☐	☐
Participating in or observing sports events	☐	☐	☐	☐	☐	☐	☐
Participating in or observing performances	☐	☐	☐	☐	☐	☐	☐
Hobbies	☐	☐	☐	☐	☐	☐	☐
Sharing meals with others	☐	☐	☐	☐	☐	☐	☐
Attending class (in person)	☐	☐	☐	☐	☐	☐	☐
Attending medical appointments	☐	☐	☐	☐	☐	☐	☐

This question lists 18 categories of life activities that are potentially affected by sound hypersensitivity. For each category, unless it is not applicable (*N/A*), the person selects *never, rarely, sometimes, often,* or *always*. In addition, the person can choose *avoid* if such activities are avoided.

Question 6 is really a follow-up to question 2 ("Is there anything you *want* to be doing, but *are not* doing because of difficulty tolerating sound?"). Both questions ask about life activities that might be affected by sound hypersensitivity. Question 2 is open-ended, which requires the person to identify any activities without being prompted with response options. The open-ended response often indicates the activity that is affected the most. Question 6 provides a fairly extensive list of categories of activities. Each category suggests different types of activities that might be affected. The combination of these two questions will identify how a person's life is actually affected. What matters most for informing treatment efforts is to understand the functional effects of the disorder. Treatment should be targeted to reducing these effects to the point where sound hypersensitivity is no longer a significant concern for the person.

Some of the 18 categories of activities in question 6 would be expected to be problematic for almost anyone and not necessarily an indication of a sound hypersensitivity disorder. Concerts are often extremely loud. Movies in a theatre may exceed safe sound intensity limits. Many religious services have loud music. Sports events are often extremely loud. If people have a problem with these types of sounds, or if they avoid them, that might be considered good sense to protect their ears. The solution in these instances is generally to wear earplugs—ideally custom-fit musician earplugs, which we'll cover in more detail in chapter 12.

Other categories are more ambiguous with respect to the level of sound experienced, which can be quite variable. These categories include shopping, restaurants, work responsibilities, driving, social activities, and hobbies. If a person has a problem with, or avoids, such activities, more information is needed to determine how loud the sounds are and if sound hypersensitivity is a factor.

For each activity reported to be a problem, it is important to understand whether the problem is one of physical discomfort, pain, emotional reactions, and/or fear. If there is any question, then one or more of the reasons listed in question 5 should be specified (*too loud, painful, annoying, make me angry, make me anxious, overwhelming, I avoid*).

7. How much time do you spend in quiet or silence?	
☐ None or very little	☐ A large amount of time
☐ A small amount	☐ Most of the time
☐ A moderate amount	☐ All of the time

People with a sound hypersensitivity disorder may tend to stay at home to avoid exposure to sound they know will be uncomfortable. Questions 5 and 6 include the response options *I avoid* and *avoid*, respectively, so it should be clear whether sound avoidance is a strategy the person uses. Question 7 puts the emphasis on such behavior to make sure the concern is adequately addressed during the interview.

The main concern is whether the person's sound-avoidance behavior is *reasonable* given the circumstances or if it might be considered *excessive*. A person may avoid being around family members or others who are eating or engaging in activities that produce sounds that trigger misophonic reactions. Misophonia is actually the concern, and such avoidance would be reasonable to preclude experiencing the reactions.

Reasonable avoidance can become excessive if a person becomes so fearful of sound that all sounds are avoided. Whether a person has crossed this threshold of "excessive" can be difficult to determine. For example, a person with pain hyperacusis may wear earplugs at home because even sounds experienced in the home are painful. For that person, the behavior is not unreasonable and therefore would not suggest phonophobia. On the other hand, a person with loudness hyperacusis may get in the habit of wearing earplugs and leave them in all day long just to avoid any chance of being exposed to uncomfortable sound. Such behavior would be excessive and would suggest the person has developed phonophobia.

It is situations like these that require judgment from a clinician who is knowledgeable about the different sound hypersensitivity disorders, how they differ, and how each is manifested. The Sound Hypersensitivity Interview can be the critical tool to obtain the information necessary to make diagnostic decisions.

---

8. Have you been diagnosed with any of these health conditions that sometimes cause difficulty tolerating sound?

☐ Post-traumatic stress disorder (PTSD) ☐ Sleep problems

☐ Anxiety disorder ☐ Depression

☐ Autism spectrum disorder ☐ Migraines

☐ Head injury (concussion, traumatic brain injury) ☐ Other_____

Question 8 provides a list of health conditions that may be linked in some way to a person's sound hypersensitivity symptoms. The link could go either way—the health condition may be the cause of the sound hypersensitivity, or the problem may worsen the health condition. Treatment would need to address both.

People who experience PTSD or autism spectrum disorder are often in a high state of alert (*hypervigilance*). Head injuries (concussion, traumatic brain injury) can also cause a state of hypervigilance. These people have heightened awareness and reactivity to sound in general—which may meet the definition of noise sensitivity. Anxiety, depression, and other psychological disorders may also have associated hypervigilance.[31] The dominant characteristic of noise sensitivity may in fact be anxiety.

Noise sensitivity is commonly experienced along with migraine headaches. According to the International Headache Society, diagnosing a migraine requires a positive response to the question, "Does light or noise bother you during a headache?"[32] Noise that is bothersome during a headache would most likely fit the definition of *loudness hyperacusis* or *noise sensitivity*.

---

9. Do you ever use earplugs or earmuffs?

☐ No → Interview is complete ☐ Yes

(If YES) What percentage of your awake time do you use earplugs or earmuffs? _____%

(If YES) Do you ever use earplugs or earmuffs in fairly quiet situations?

☐ No ☐ Yes

Is this a situation of overprotecting ears due to problems with sound tolerance?

☐ No ☐ Yes

If the person wears earplugs or earmuffs, two additional questions are asked to determine whether *overprotecting* the ears is a concern. People of course need to be aware that loud sound can cause inner ear damage and worsen any sound hypersensitivity—thus necessitating the appropriate use of hearing protection. They also need to know, however, that *inappropriate* use of hearing protection can worsen sound hypersensitivity.

Some people use earplugs or earmuffs because of their belief that certain sounds, or sound in general, will cause their tinnitus or sound hypersensitivity to become worse. They need to be educated that *overuse* of hearing protection can result in heightened sensitivity to sound.[33] If such overuse has already occurred, then it is important that the person take steps to reverse any heightened sensitivity by gradually reducing the use of hearing protection. They need to progress to the point of only using hearing protection when exposed to sounds that can cause damage to the auditory system.

The concern for overprotection may not apply to people with pain hyperacusis. For these people, *any* sound may cause burning, stabbing, jabbing pain.[5,6] They may need to wear earplugs/earmuffs all day long. That would not be a case of overprotecting the ears—it would just be doing whatever is necessary to survive in a world of painful sound. It is critical that the clinician is aware of this population without assuming that every person with hyperacusis should wean off of hearing protection and gradually be exposed to more and more sound in order to desensitize the auditory system. We will have much more to say about pain hyperacusis in chapter 7.

Summary

We've covered every question from the Sound Hypersensitivity Interview. The intent of each question is explained and examples are provided for what different responses might suggest. The dynamics of conducting the Interview are nuanced and dependent on the skill and knowledge of the examiner. The point of conducting the Interview is to gain an understanding of exactly how a person is hypersensitive to sound, what diagnosis might be appropriate, and whether treatment is warranted.

The Interview should be administered only if a person has indicated a sound hypersensitivity problem that is not confused with hearing aids being too loud, reacting to sound that really *is* too loud, or just being annoyed by certain sounds that would be annoying to almost anyone.

Proper screening should rule out these sorts of confusions to ensure that anyone who completes the Interview really does have a sound hypersensitivity problem that needs to be formally evaluated.

A common scenario for a person with a sound hyper-sensitivity complaint is to meet with an audiologist. The audiologist completes a medical history, brief tinnitus evaluation (if tinnitus is present), hearing assessment, and screening for sound hypersensitivity. If the person screens positive for sound hypersensitivity, that would suggest the need to conduct the Sound Hypersensitivity Interview. Because the Interview can require up to an hour to thoroughly and carefully cover each question, a separate appointment might be necessary.

The information obtained by the audiologist sets the stage for completing the Interview and then making a diagnosis. The next five chapters address diagnosis, and a chapter is devoted to each of the five disorders. At the beginning of each chapter, a working definition is provided for the disorder covered by that chapter. Chapters 11–16 describe the treatment methods that are available to treat each of the disorders.

PART 3

Diagnosing Sound Hypersensitivity Disorders

CHAPTER 6

Diagnosing Loudness Hyperacusis

Working Definition of Loudness Hyperacusis

Loudness hyperacusis is the experience of uncomfortable-to-unbearable physical sensations (exclusive of piercing, burning, or stabbing pain) in the ears and/or head when exposed to any sound at intensity levels that are comfortable for most people.

This definition is the basis for making a diagnosis of loudness hyperacusis, which is characterized by a person's inability to tolerate the loudness of sounds that are easily tolerated by the average person. Loudness hyperacusis involves often indescribable sensations of physical discomfort in the ears and/or head that would not be described as "burning, stabbing, jabbing pain." Some of the sensations might involve an unpleasant sense of fullness in one or both ears (like a balloon being blown up inside the ear), dull earache, or headache.

Any of these characteristic physical sensations of loudness hyperacusis would meet some definitions of pain. For purposes of diagnosing a sound hypersensitivity disorder, however, it is critical to use this working definition because loudness hyperacusis is very different from pain hyperacusis. Pain hyperacusis is distinguished by *burning, stabbing, jabbing pain*, while loudness hyperacusis is characterized by *uncomfortable-to-unbearable physical sensations*.

Why "uncomfortable-to-unbearable"? These words describe a range of sound-induced discomfort that would be on a continuum from *mildly uncomfortable* to *moderately uncomfortable* to *unbearable*. The actual physical sensation is difficult to put into words without using the word *pain*. The word pain, however, needs to be reserved to describe the burning, stabbing, jabbing pain that would be the hallmark of pain hyperacusis.

How Physical Discomfort Is Described

How do people with loudness hyperacusis describe the physical discomfort they experience? It is not uncommon that they have trouble describing the symptoms and will default to using the word *pain*. When this occurs, it is essential to precisely define the word pain to differentiate between pain hyperacusis and loudness hyperacusis. The definition of pain in the context of pain hyperacusis is provided in the next chapter, Diagnosing Pain Hyperacusis.

The following descriptions of loudness hyperacusis are representative of what can be found in the scientific literature.

- "experience of inordinate loudness of sound"[34]
- "the perception of everyday environmental sound as being overwhelmingly loud or intense"[24]
- "everyday sounds being perceived as intense and overwhelming"[19]
- "when sound is of a moderate intensity it is perceived as loud and intrusive"[19]
- "abnormally strong reaction to sound, occurring within the auditory pathways, in levels that would not trouble a normal individual"[12]

A research group reviewed 43 studies that were published about hyperacusis to help guide future hyperacusis research.[24] Of these 43 studies, 29 provided "a working definition of hyperacusis." Some of those definitions that are most relevant to loudness hyperacusis are the following:

- "reduced sound tolerance"
- "lowered threshold for sound tolerance"
- "a reduction of normal tolerance for everyday sounds"
- "intolerance to the loudness of sounds that most individuals deem to be tolerable"
- "unusual hypersensitivity or discomfort induced by exposure to sound"
- "oversensitivity to sound"
- "an increased sensitivity to auditory stimulation"

It should be noted that these descriptions might also be made by people with *noise sensitivity*, which is a different disorder (chapter 9). It can be difficult to distinguish between loudness hyperacusis and noise sensitivity.

Loudness hyperacusis is physical discomfort that occurs whenever any sound reaches a certain intensity level. Noise sensitivity is an emotional response to sound in general, often described as "feeling overwhelmed."

Different Degrees of Loudness Hyperacusis

In chapter 4, a rough guide to diagnosing a mild, moderate, severe, or extreme sound hypersensitivity disorder is suggested. We will now apply that guide to different degrees of loudness hyperacusis.

Mild Loudness Hyperacusis

A *mild* case of loudness hyperacusis would mean a person has "minimal but significant interference with normal life activities" (chapter 4). Some sounds are uncomfortably loud but are not experienced often. The person might have physical discomfort when in crowded places such as shopping centers, restaurants, and parties. Other types of sounds may cause discomfort, such as clattering dishes, some traffic noises, and musical performances. The sounds may be uncomfortably loud to the person, but tolerable.

Moderate Loudness Hyperacusis

Moderate loudness hyperacusis would cause "substantial interference with normal life activities" (chapter 4). This person is bothered by more types of sounds and more often than the person with mild loudness hyperacusis. When bothered, the person with moderate loudness hyperacusis may feel the urge to leave the premises or wear earplugs. Leaving the premises can be socially awkward, and wearing earplugs may be the only acceptable means to tolerate these uncomfortable surroundings (although inserting and wearing earplugs may attract unwanted attention). The frequent use of earplugs can result in the person becoming overly dependent on them, resulting in overprotection of the ears and potentially worsening the loudness tolerance problem.[33]

Severe or Extreme Loudness Hyperacusis

Severe loudness hyperacusis causes "extensive interference with normal life activities" (chapter 4). *Extreme* loudness hyperacusis "prevents some or all normal life activities." All of the concerns described for moderate loudness hyperacusis exist for the person who is severely/extremely afflicted but to a much greater degree. This person is bothered by sounds at low levels and may wear earplugs and/or earmuffs almost continually—especially outside of the home. These behaviors also describe severe pain hyperacusis, and so the distinction between loudness hyperacusis and pain hyperacusis is critical to ensure that treatment recommendations are appropriate. Other than making that distinction, it is relatively straightforward to diagnose a person with severe/extreme loudness hyperacusis. Such a person tends to avoid any noisy situation, wears earplugs/earmuffs all or most of the time, and cannot participate in many or all of the normal activities of life.

Is There an Emotional Component?

According to our working definition of loudness hyperacusis, the disorder is limited to the physical discomfort that is experienced in reaction to sound. The physical discomfort is what defines loudness hyperacusis and is the reason for the diagnosis. Importantly, the physical discomfort can be accompanied by emotional reactions. These reactions would be considered secondary to the primary complaint, but they need to be taken into account when planning treatment.

We might think of two versions of a loudness hyperacusis disorder—one with an emotional component and one without an emotional component. In both cases, the physical discomfort is the symptom that should be the primary focus of treatment. We operate on the assumption that the disorder is due to enhanced auditory gain (as explained in appendix F). If there is an emotional component, the emotions should be treated separately from the loudness hyperacusis—while recognizing that *the emotions are reactions to the physical discomfort.*

Whether the loudness hyperacusis is mild, moderate, severe, or extreme, the diagnosis should take into account any emotional reactions identified during the Sound Hypersensitivity Interview (chapter 5). Addressing associated emotional reactions should be part of the treatment plan and may require additional assessment for possible anxiety and depression. Because emotional distress can cause sleep disruption, the possibility of insomnia should also be assessed.

What Causes Loudness Hyperacusis?

Appendix F contains a description of *central auditory gain,* which is the "volume control" for our auditory system. There is "extensive evidence" that central auditory gain is increased following damage to the cochlea.[35]

Briefly, all of the neurons in the central auditory system fire spontaneously—even when there is no sound. The spontaneous activity has a "set-point," which is recalibrated depending on the level of sound entering the ears.[35,36] During an extended period of quiet, for example, the set-point may be raised such that the central auditory system amplifies sound more than usual, which could result in loudness hyperacusis. "A consensus is emerging in the auditory neuroscience literature that hyperacusis may be associated with a sustained and persistent increase in central auditory gain."[24] (p. 2)

Another source of physical discomfort can be caused by tightening of the *tensor tympani muscle*—one of the two middle ear muscles that contract to stiffen the middle ear bones (ossicles), which reduces the amount of sound energy entering the cochlea. Physical discomfort associated with loudness hyperacusis could be due to everyday sounds causing contraction of the tensor tympani muscle, which would cause a sensation of fullness in the ear and other uncomfortable sensations. Some people have *tensor tympani syndrome,* which could explain why the tensor tympani contracts so easily with sound exposure. The tensor tympani muscle and tensor tympani syndrome are more fully described in appendix E.

Additional Considerations

Although the definition of loudness hyperacusis refers specifically to physical discomfort, "there is undoubtedly an emotional and psychological component."[19] (p. 358) It is therefore important to evaluate how loudness hyperacusis affects the person emotionally and ensure that any significant emotional reactions are properly addressed.

In the scientific literature, sound hypersensitivity that coincides with migraine headache is referred to as *phonophobia*.[32] This coincident sound hypersensitivity would most likely actually be *loudness hyperacusis* or *noise sensitivity*. Phonophobia, according to how it is defined in this book, refers specifically to the excessive and persistent fear of sound. Appendix E contains more information about migraine and sound hypersensitivity.

Lastly, loudness hyperacusis is almost always bilateral (experienced in both ears or both sides of the head).[19] Also, most people with hyperacusis prefer to be in a quiet environment, even if they have tinnitus.

CHAPTER 7

Diagnosing Pain Hyperacusis

Working Definition of Pain Hyperacusis

Pain hyperacusis (noxacusis) is the experience of burning, stabbing, or jabbing pain in the ears or head when exposed to, and/or following, any sound at an intensity level that would be comfortable for most people.

Healthcare professionals do not widely recognize pain hyperacusis.[37] "The old way of thinking is that there is one kind of hyperacusis, where everything sounds louder. Fortunately, science has progressed, and it's now known that there is a more severe form, pain hyperacusis, where loudness passes some threshold and turns into actual pain. And that pain lingers and worsens. It's impossible to describe how much suffering this condition entails."[6] (p. 32)

How do we determine "where loudness passes some threshold and turns into actual pain"? This is difficult to

61

determine because much of what can be said about loud-ness hyperacusis also pertains to pain hyperacusis. "Some individuals perceive everyday sounds to be excessively loud (i.e., *loudness hyperacusis*), whereas others experience physical pain in response to sounds (i.e., *pain hyperacusis* or *noxacusis*)."[37] [(p. 2)] The key is to determine what is unique about pain hyperacusis that makes it an exclusive disorder. The most important concern is to know how *pain* is defined.

How Pain Is Described for Pain Hyperacusis

To address how pain is defined for pain hyperacusis, we'll go straight to the most credible sources—descriptions by people who experience pain hyperacusis and professionals who work with these people.

- "Almost any audible sound now causes pain—it feels like burning acid being poured into my ears, or a severe sunburn in my ear canals."[6]
- "It felt like someone stabbing my ear with a knife."[6]
- "debilitating sound-induced pain"[37]
- "a burning, aching fullness deep within my ears that can last for days or weeks"[38]
- "excruciating pain that can last for weeks or months"[37]
- "point of pain deep within the ear canal"[6]
- "stabbing pain through my ears"[6]
- "a deep burning sensation"[6]
- "the sound of running water was painful"[38]
- "a burning, stabbing, jabbing pain that feels like someone is pushing hot pokers into their ears"[5]

- "sound-induced burning, stabbing, throbbing, and pinching that occurs either in the ear or elsewhere in the body (i.e., referred pain)"[37]
- "it is a real pain condition.... Another thing we don't understand is the delayed reaction we see with pain hyperacusis."[5]

Other Unique Features

In addition to their distinctive descriptions of pain, people with pain hyperacusis seem to have the most severe form of hyperacusis; they experience "setbacks," sound therapy is ineffective, and the pain may be delayed and/or prolonged. These features are recognized by researchers as revealed by the following quotes.

- "What nobody understands is that the noise is not just painful in the moment. Too much exposure to this kind of noise causes a setback—increased sensitivity and a burning, aching fullness deep within my ears that can last for days or weeks."[38]
- "People with loudness hyperacusis are bothered and might even feel pain, but it is not debilitating. They don't have the same type of pain as individuals with pain hyperacusis, and they don't have setbacks."[5]
- "People with loudness hyperacusis even say things like, 'When I go in the kitchen I just tough it out.' People with pain hyperacusis cannot tough it out."[5]
- "Individuals with pain hyperacusis often.... report frequent 'setbacks' (i.e., symptom exacerbations in

response to a trigger sound) and reduced benefit from behavioral interventions (e.g., sound therapy)."[37]

- "The pain often fluctuates in severity, location, and quality, and it can occur immediately after a sound exposure, or it can be delayed by several hours."[37]

What Causes Pain Hyperacusis?

This question is addressed in some detail in appendix G. As discussed above, and in appendix F, loudness hyperacusis is thought to be a condition caused by an increase in central auditory gain. That would not be the case for pain hyperacusis. "There is little-to-no empirical evidence to support central gain as the underlying cause of pain hyperacusis per se."[37]

Very briefly, pain hyperacusis may be caused primarily by neurons that connect the outer hair cells in the cochlea to the brain stem, via the auditory nerve.[7] These type II neurons have the same properties as C-fibers that are pain receptors (nociceptors) in the skin. "Liu et al. (2015)[39] demonstrated that type II afferent neural fibers terminating on the outer hair cells were selectively activated when hair cell damage occurred in the cochlea. These type II fibers activated neurons in the cochlear nucleus when damaging sounds were subsequently presented to the cochlea, and Flores et al. (2015)[40] proposed activation of these type II nerve fibers might serve as a mechanism for pain hyperacusis."[41] (p. 20)

Other possible mechanisms for sound-induced pain include structures in the middle ear and central auditory pathway.[37] In the middle ear, damage, overload, or myoclonus (uncontrollable twitching) of the tensor tympani muscle (appendix E) can irritate the trigeminal nerve (appendix G), resulting in pain in or near the ear. Regarding the central auditory pathway, damage to the middle or inner ear can lead to an increase in neural activity. Evidence for any of these theories is based largely on theory or animal models. "Taken together with existing theories and other surveys of pain hyperacusis, we feel that our results are most consistent with trigeminal nerve involvement."[37] (p. 18)

Summary

Both loudness hyperacusis and pain hyperacusis are defined by physical reactions to sound at intensity levels that would not be uncomfortable for most people. The main distinction is how the physical reactions are described. For loudness hyperacusis, they are described as intolerance, hypersensitivity, discomfort, etc. Pain hyperacusis is described as burning, stabbing, jabbing, sharp, excruciating, burning acid, stabbing knife, hot pokers, etc. Pain hyperacusis also results in delayed or prolonged pain.

The distinctions can be difficult to make because of how people describe their symptoms. Use of the word *pain* can be a source of confusion, requiring clarification to know exactly what is meant by the individual. It can be helpful to think of loudness hyperacusis as a disorder caused by increased auditory gain, and pain hyperacusis as caused by pain receptors in or near the ear. Pain hyperacusis would also be a generally more severe disorder than loudness hyperacusis.

CHAPTER 8

Diagnosing Misophonia

Misophonia is characterized by strong negative emotional responses (anger, irritation, disgust, anxiety, rage), physiological responses (increased muscular tension, increased heart rate, sweating), and behavioral responses (agitation, aggression) to "trigger" sounds (most often made by the mouth and nose; also other human-made sounds, sounds of objects like ticking clocks, animal sounds) and occasionally visual triggers (jiggling or swinging legs, watching someone eat).

This is a rather lengthy definition, which is necessary because of the complexity of the disorder. The definition is derived from the *consensus definition of misophonia*.

Consensus Definition of Misophonia

Misophonia was first named and described in the scientific literature in 2002.[42] The disorder was recognized by various healthcare fields but without an agreed-upon definition. This lack of agreement motivated an effort to establish a "consensus definition of misophonia," which was completed and published in 2022.[43] A *modified Delphi method*[23] was used to achieve the consensus definition (as described in appendix D). The consensus definition is copied verbatim below (all in *italics*).

General Description

"Misophonia is a disorder of decreased tolerance to specific sounds or stimuli associated with such sounds. These stimuli, known as 'triggers,' are experienced as unpleasant or distressing and tend to evoke strong negative emotional, physiological, and behavioral responses that are not seen in most other people. Misophonic responses do not seem be elicited by the loudness of auditory stimuli, but rather by the specific pattern or meaning to an individual. Trigger stimuli are often repetitive and primarily, but not exclusively, include stimuli generated by another individual, especially those produced by the human body. Once a trigger stimulus is detected, individuals with misophonia may have difficulty distracting themselves from the stimulus and may experience suffering, distress, and/or impairment in social, occupational, or academic functioning. The expression of misophonic symptoms varies, as does the severity, which ranges from mild to severe impairments. Some individuals with misophonia

are aware that their reactions to misophonic trigger stimuli are disproportionate to the circumstances. Misophonia symptoms are typically first observed in childhood or early adolescence.

Reactions to Misophonic Triggers

In response to specific trigger stimuli, individuals with misophonia may experience a range of negative affective reactions. Anger, irritation, disgust, and anxiety are most common, though some individuals may experience rage. Misophonic triggers may evoke increased autonomic arousal such as increased muscular tension, increased heart rate, and sweating.

Trigger stimuli may also evoke strong behavioral reactions such as agitation or aggression directed toward the individual producing the stimulus. On rare occasions, aggression may be expressed as verbal or physical outbursts although these responses are seen more in children with misophonia than in adults. Individuals with misophonia often engage in behaviors to mitigate their reactions to triggers such as: avoiding or escaping from situations in which they encounter trigger stimuli; seeking to discontinue the triggering stimuli; mimicking or reproducing the triggers.

Influences on Reactions

The strength of an individual's reaction to a misophonic trigger stimulus may be influenced by multiple factors including but not limited to: the context in which the stimulus is encountered; the individual's perceived degree of control over the stimulus source; and the interpersonal relationship between the individual with misophonia and the source of the trigger. Self-generated stimuli typically do not evoke the same aversive responses as stimuli produced by other people.

Functional Impairments

Individuals' reactions to misophonia triggers may cause significant distress, interfere with day-to-day life, and may contribute to mental health problems. Individuals with misophonia may experience functional impairments that range from mild to severe including but not limited to impaired occupational and/or academic functioning, concentration difficulties, and an inability to perform important work tasks. Individuals may also experience impaired social functioning, strained social relationships, and social isolation resulting from their misophonia symptoms.

Relationship to Other Conditions/Disorders

Misophonia can be present in people with or without normal hearing thresholds, and can occur alone or with the auditory conditions of tinnitus and hyperacusis. Misophonia can also occur with neurological or psychiatric conditions or disorders including but not limited to: anxiety disorders, mood disorders, personality disorders, obsessive compulsive related disorders, post-traumatic stress disorder, autism spectrum disorder, attention deficit hyperactivity disorder. For any given individual, the symptoms of misophonia should not be better explained by any co-occurring disorders.

Misophonic Triggers

Although each person may have their own pattern of triggers, some stimuli serve as common misophonic triggers. Auditory triggers are most common, although individuals with miso-phonia may also identify distress in response to visual triggers.

Sounds associated with oral functions are among the most often reported misophonic trigger stimuli, such as chewing, eating, smacking lips, slurping, coughing, throat clearing, and swallowing. Nasal sounds, such as breathing and sniffing, often serve as triggers as well. Auditory triggers may also include non-oral/nasal sounds produced by people such as pen clicking, keyboard typing, finger or foot tapping and shuffling footsteps, as well as sounds produced by objects, such as a clock ticking, or sound generated by animals. Visual triggers have been reported to include stimuli such as cracking knuckles and jiggling or swinging legs, as well as visual stimuli associated with an auditory trigger, such as watching someone eat."[43] (pp. 10-12)

Most Common Symptoms of Misophonia

The Misophonia Consensus Committee provided a valuable service by publishing their consensus definition.[43] The publication is available on the internet as a free download. Their definition is so complete that little can be added that would contribute significantly. We can, however, include a few quotes from various authors that reflect what is most commonly experienced with misophonia—*strong negative emotions that are triggered by oral and nasal sounds.*

- "Misophonia is defined as an abnormally intense reaction to breathing, coughing, throat clearing, food chewing, crunching, swallowing, lip-smacking, spitting, and similar sounds.... symptoms range from disgust, distress, and discomfort, to irritation, anger, hatred, fear, and annoyance."[44]

- "an acquired aversive reaction to specific human generated sounds such as eating sound or breathing, the response being characterized by anger and sometimes rage"[24]
- "an aversive reaction to specific 'trigger' sounds characterized by anger, extreme annoyance, and disgust"[3]
- "Strong emotions such as anger, irritation, disgust, or anxiety are evoked immediately when people with misophonia hear particular sounds."[10]

Misophonia Questionnaires

Along with other sound hypersensitivity questionnaires, questionnaires for assessing misophonia are summarized in appendix B. One of those questionnaires is the Amsterdam Misophonia Scale. A study that evaluated the Amsterdam Misophonia Scale proposed the presence of at least four of five possible symptoms "as a decisive measure for high perceived misophonia."[44] The five possible symptoms include:

1. Irritation or anger against people making trigger sounds
2. Strong wish to react against people making trigger sounds
3. Feeling of imminent loss of self-control
4. Feeling of excessive anger
5. Interference with social functioning

Each of the misophonia questionnaires reviewed in appendix B has unique characteristics. Any of them can be useful in the process of diagnosing misophonia, while bearing in mind that different questionnaires will result in different outcomes.

What Causes Misophonia?

Misophonia is a complex disorder with an unknown cause.[45] It is debated whether it is an auditory disorder or a psychiatric disorder.[46] Although misophonia is triggered by sounds, the condition is independent of auditory function—people with normal hearing, hearing loss, and various auditory disorders can experience misophonia.[45] The negative experience also does not activate the auditory system—it activates emotional areas of the brain.

It has been proposed that misophonia is the result of the limbic system and autonomic nervous system reacting "abnormally to auditory input of normal intensity."[45] (p. 7) These systems are areas of the brain that are activated when a sound carries emotional significance.[27] The *limbic system* underlies emotions. Its connections with the auditory nervous system are the means for sounds to evoke emotional responses when the sounds are associated with certain memories.

The *autonomic nervous system* controls basic bodily functions such as breathing, heartbeat, blood pressure, sweating, and many others.[27] Misophonic trigger sounds can cause the sympathetic part of the autonomic nervous system to become strongly activated, resulting in adrenaline release into the bloodstream, increased heart rate, shortness of breath, increased muscle tension, and distress.[45] Various other brain areas have been shown to become overactivated for people with misophonia when exposed to trigger sounds.[44]

Symptoms of misophonia often start during childhood or early adolescence.[45] One study reported the average age in its patients that misophonia started was 13 years.[46] Its onset "may be associated with unpleasant childhood memories of sounds emitted by family members (e.g., during meals)."[45] (p. 6) More generally, its onset is associated with some triggering event that evokes unpleasant emotions such as disgust. This may be due to the presence of other disorders that predispose the person to be triggered by certain sounds. It is unclear whether trauma can explain the onset of symptoms.

A correlation has been shown between obsessive-compulsive personality disorder (OCPD) and misophonia.[46] "People with misophonia show characteristics of OCPD." (p. 3) Being preoccupied with certain trigger sounds resembles the *obsessionality* (being obsessional) that is characteristic of obsessive-compulsive disorder (OCD). (Note that obsessions are a diagnostic criterion for OCD but not for OCPD. Also, OCD is an anxiety disorder whereas OCPD is not an anxiety disorder). "The symptoms, personality traits, and coping mechanisms of the patients showed a striking similarity in nature and development. The consistent pattern of symptoms suggested the presence of a discrete and independent disorder."[46] (p. 1)

"Whether misophonia should be classified as a discrete psychiatric disorder is still a matter of debate. Misophonia is often associated with symptoms of other psychological disorders, predominantly with anxiety and depression. Furthermore, misophonia shares some similarities with obsessive-compulsive disorder, but differs from it in the reaction to the stimuli. Misophonia symptoms were also reportedly associated with post-traumatic stress disorder, attention-deficit disorder, eating disorders, selective mutism, etc."[44] (p. 45)

Evidence for the genetic predisposition to develop misophonia has been provided in studies showing that multiple members of the same family had misophonia and that a high percentage of people with misophonia reported a family history having the same symptoms.[45] It is possible that children learn the behaviors of family members, although some children acquire the symptoms even with little family contact.

Summary

Although the word misophonia literally means *hate sound*, this "translation is misleading, because the essence of the condition is selective sound aversion, not a hypersensitivity to all kinds of sounds."[10] (p. 447) The disorder can involve reactions to visual stimuli, but they are predominantly triggered by sounds—most commonly oral and nasal sounds.

Other sounds that have been suggested as possible trigger sounds include kissing, finger tapping, nail clipping, footsteps, keyboard typing, pen clicking, glasses clinking, rustling of paper or plastic, loud human voices, babies crying, noisy neighbors, traffic, household appliances, dogs barking, and claws clicking.[44] Clearly, some of these sounds may just reflect common annoyance from everyday sounds, as explained in chapter 3. It is always essential to conduct a comprehensive assessment to avoid misdiagnosing misophonia based on common annoyance.

CHAPTER 9

Diagnosing Noise Sensitivity

Working Definition of Noise Sensitivity

Noise sensitivity is hypersensitivity to usual sounds that are interpreted as unwanted "noise" and cause annoyance, tension, anxiety, fear, isolation tendency, and/or anger, which may be accompanied by physical reactions such as irregular heartbeat.

"Noise sensitivity implies a trait present to some degree in everyone, accentuated in some people and less prominent in others. It is thus expected to vary normally within a healthy population."[47] (p. 8) To paraphrase that quote, *noise sensitivity is a universal trait because everyone is annoyed by some sounds* (as explained in chapter 3). Diagnosing a noise sensitivity *disorder* therefore requires determining whether the person's life is *significantly impacted* because of noise sensitivity. Further, it is necessary to differentiate noise sensitivity from the other sound hypersensitivity disorders when there are likely overlapping symptoms.

For example, "noise sensitivity and hyperacusis are not always explicitly defined in papers, which contributes to the confusion between the two terms.... both conditions include auditory symptoms that may involve overlapping manifestations such as avoidance of sound/noise, the use of ear protection, and anxiety."[48] (p. 2) Another group wrote, "Hyperacusis is considered upfront as a pathological auditory condition with a putative cause (i.e., etiology) or an underlying biological dysfunction, rather than a symptom present to some degree in all individuals. In other words, whereas everyone experiences 'some degree' of noise sensitivity, not everyone should experience 'some degree' of hyperacusis."[47] (p. 8)

Any confusion between noise sensitivity and hyperacusis would pertain to loudness hyperacusis, not pain hyperacusis. With loudness hyperacusis, physical discomfort is experienced when any sound reaches a certain intensity level. Noise sensitivity does not involve physical discomfort—the reactions to sound are, by definition, negative emotions.

Noise sensitivity can also be confused with misophonia because both are characterized by emotional reactions to sound. "Noise sensitivity and misophonia could be related through neuroticism as a common feature."[44] (p. 45) Neuroticism refers to emotional ups and downs and can include anxiety, depression, irritability, moodiness, and a low tolerance for stress.[26,49] The main distinction is that misophonia involves reactions to *certain sounds* while noise sensitivity involves reactions to *sound in general*. "Unlike misophonia, noise sensitivity is not related to any specific sound, but rather to the attitudes toward unwanted sound in various situations."[44] (p. 41)

Making the diagnosis can depend partly on completion of a noise sensitivity questionnaire (see appendix B). Ultimately, however, an interview such as the Sound Hypersensitivity Interview (chapter 5) is necessary to identify symptoms that would support the diagnosis and differentiate noise sensitivity from other sound hypersensitivity disorders.

A standardized protocol for assessing noise sensitivity has not been developed.[50] Using the Sound Hypersensitivity Interview will help disentangle the characteristic symptoms from effects of mood, cognitive deficits, and personality disorders—all of which are associated with noise sensitivity. Clearly, anxiety alone induces noise sensitivity, and depression may have the same effect. The dominant characteristic of noise sensitivity may in fact be anxiety, which increases sensory sensitivity overall (*hypervigilance/ hyperarousal*).[31] Diagnosing noise sensitivity therefore might benefit from the use of anxiety measures.[50] For example, the Hospital Anxiety and Depression Scale (HADS) is well known for assessing both anxiety and depression.[51]

Unique Characteristics of Noise Sensitivity

In chapter 1, it's explained that much of the information in this book is derived from peer-reviewed articles that were identified by searching on PubMed. At the time of this writing, there were almost 100 peer-reviewed articles about noise sensitivity indexed in PubMed. After reviewing many of these it was clear that noise sensitivity is fairly consistently defined in the scientific literature. Below are some quotes that describe how noise sensitivity is a unique disorder.

- "Noise sensitivity.... has been used to differentiate people with a strong dislike of noise from those who are indifferent to noise or who are not bothered at all by noise."[48]
- "Noise sensitive individuals are likely to pay more attention to sound and evaluate it negatively, to have stronger emotional reactions to noise, and greater difficulty habituating."[47]
- "Among individuals exposed to the same noise, those with high noise sensitivity are more likely to pay attention to the noise, to interpret the noise negatively as a threat or annoyance, and to react emotionally, compared to those with low noise sensitivity. Consequently, it is difficult for those with high noise sensitivity to become habituated to noise."[52]
- "Students who are sensitive to noise perform worse in academic ability, are more uneasy in interpersonal communication, and have a stronger desire for privacy."[53]
- "increased reactivity to sounds that may include general discomfort (annoyance or feeling overwhelmed) due to a perceived noisy environment, regardless of its loudness"[4]
- "mild anger, partly as a result of noise interference into everyday activities, coupled with feelings of invasion of privacy, and lack of control"[48]

Some articles point out how noise sensitivity is an emotional disorder that is independent of the loudness and other characteristics of sound and, more generally, of auditory system functioning.

- "Noise sensitivity is predicated on noise annoyance, a negative emotional response to noise; it was shown—in survey/modeling studies—to be only slightly correlated or even unrelated to noise levels."[47]
- "does not seem to be related to abnormalities in the peripheral auditory system"[48]
- "there is no significant relation between auditory thresholds as measured by an audiometer and subjective noise sensitivity."[54]
- "noise sensitivity—a stable trait that is independent of noise exposure"[52]

Studies also focus on how environmental noise ultimately can have negative effects on physical and mental health.

- "Individuals with high noise sensitivity are more likely to experience physical or mental diseases."[52]
- "There is recent evidence that noise sensitivity may be a moderator of the effects of environmental noise on physical ill-health, for instance, cardiovascular outcomes and possibly more likely, psychological ill-health."[48]
- "negative emotions including fear and anger, accompanied by physiological arousal, which reinforces initial affective reactions, leading to negative health effects"[55]
- "consistent predictor of depressive symptoms and psychological distress"[52]

Noise Sensitivity Questionnaires

Appendix B describes two questionnaires that have been developed and validated for assessing noise sensitivity. These include the Noise Sensitivity Scale[56] and the Noise Sensitivity Questionnaire.[57] The most widely used is the Noise Sensitivity Scale, which has 21 questions that ask about general attitudes toward noise and how noise causes annoyance or distress.[47] The Noise Sensitivity Questionnaire contains 35 questions that ask how noise affects five areas of daily life: leisure, work, habitation, communication, and sleep. Both of these questionnaires are limited to distinguishing between low-, medium-, and high-noise-sensitive individuals. They are not intended to be used to diagnose a noise sensitivity disorder but would be helpful in making the diagnosis.

What Causes Noise Sensitivity?

This is a difficult question to answer because of the numerous possible factors that can be involved. Appendix H addresses this question. Briefly, it is often thought that personality traits are a major factor. Personality traits that have been linked to noise sensitivity include anxiety, depression, introversion, extraversion, and conscientiousness. In addition, people with post-traumatic stress disorder (PTSD) may experience *hypervigilance* (or *hyperarousal*) to all environmental stimuli, including sounds.[58,59]

Neuronal mechanisms in the brain have been proposed to underlie noise sensitivity.[54,60] Changes that occur in the cortex as well as other areas of the brain have been implicated.[44,53,60] Other studies have revealed a genetic basis of noise sensitivity.[48,54]

Summary

Everyone is annoyed by some sounds, but that does not mean they have a sound hypersensitivity disorder. To diagnose noise sensitivity, the person should have a problem that would be described by our working definition for noise sensitivity (at the beginning of this chapter), and the problem should have at least a "minimal but significant interference with normal life activities" (see chapter 4). Importantly, fulfilling the description of the working definition is less important than the degree to which the disorder impacts the person's life.

CHAPTER 10

Diagnosing Phonophobia

Phonophobia is an excessive, persistent state of fear that either specific sounds or sound in general will cause discomfort, distress, or pain.

Definition of Phobia

Phonophobia has different meanings depending on context. Most generally, "a phobia is a persistent, excessive, unrealistic fear of an object, person, animal, activity, or situation. It is a type of anxiety disorder. A person with a phobia either tries to avoid the thing that triggers the fear, or endures it with great anxiety and distress."[14]

This general definition of *phobia* applies perfectly to phonophobia—just change the definition slightly to: "*Phonophobia* is a persistent, excessive, unrealistic fear of *sound*.

It is a type of anxiety disorder. A person with *phonophobia* either tries to avoid the *sound* that triggers the fear, or endures it with great anxiety and distress."

A *specific phobia* refers to excessive fear associated with a specific object or situation (*sound* in the case of phonophobia). "People who suffer from specific phobias work hard to avoid their phobia stimuli even though they know there is no threat or danger, but they feel powerless."[61] (p. 462)

DSM-5 Criteria for a Specific Phobia Diagnosis

The American Psychiatric Association publishes the Diagnostic and Statistical Manual of Mental Disorders. The DSM-5 is the fifth edition of the manual.[62] According to the DSM-5, criteria that must be met to diagnose a specific phobia include "excessive fear, and immediate anxiety response, and avoidance of the fear trigger. Such symptoms must limit a person's ability to function, last at least six months, and not be due to another mental disorder."[15]

Definitions of Phonophobia in the Scientific Literature

When using the term *phobia* in relation to *sound*, there are different perspectives. In the scientific literature, the term *phonophobia* typically refers to some form of sound hypersensitivity as a symptom of migraine headache. In fact, in 2004 the International Headache Society stated that diagnosing a migraine required phonophobia (and/or *photophobia*—hypersensitivity to light) being reported in response to the question, "Does light or noise bother you during a headache?"[32] Noise that is bothersome during a headache would most likely fit our working definitions of *loudness hyperacusis* (chapter 6) or *noise sensitivity* (chapter 9). Phonophobia, according to how it is defined in this chapter, refers specifically to the excessive fear of sound—not reactions to sound.

Chapter 1 contains a description of PubMed and how it has been used as a source to find peer-reviewed articles that support what is written in this book. A PubMed search for "phonophobia" as a word in the title of articles resulted in only 26 publications. Of these, most describe phonophobia as a symptom of migraine headache. There are very few publications that focus on phonophobia as the type of disorder that meets our working definition. A few authors describe phonophobia in a manner that is consistent with our working definition, as quoted below.

- "a persistent, abnormal, and unwarranted fear of sound"[12]
- "a persistent, abnormal, and unwarranted fear of certain sounds"[3]
- "a specific phobia of certain sounds or sound sources"[63]
- "a specific phobia of certain sounds or categories of sounds"[64]
- "sounds are innocuous to most people, yet provoke fear in others"[9]

These definitions are still not entirely consistent. For example, does phonophobia mean fear of *all* sounds, or fear of *certain* sounds or *categories* of sounds? Answer: It depends on the underlying sound hypersensitivity disorder. People have phonophobia because of sound being physically or emotionally bothersome, meaning they have loudness hyperacusis, pain hyperacusis, misophonia, and/or noise sensitivity. If a person has loudness hyperacusis, pain hyperacusis, or noise sensitivity, then the fear would be of sound in general (because these are disorders that pertain to *all* sounds). If the person has misophonia, then the fear would be of certain sounds or categories of sound (specific sounds that cause emotional reactions). These principles are of course generalizations, and there are exceptions.

Healthy Fear of Sound

Is it possible to fear sound in a healthy way? Actually, yes. "Fear is an emotion of anticipation that is triggered when a situation that is at risk for our safety.... is perceived."[61] (p. 462) Note that fear pertains to *anticipation* of a threatening event and not *reacting* to the event. Fear helps *prepare* the body to face a potentially dangerous situation. That kind of fear is normal and *healthy*.

People with symptoms of sound hypersensitivity take normal precautions to keep from being exposed to sound they know will be uncomfortable (too loud, painful, emotion-triggering, and/or annoying). *Normal precautions* would typically involve wearing earplugs or earmuffs, or avoiding the offending sound altogether. These would be reasonable actions to take to avoid discomfort.

Anyone with a sound hypersensitivity disorder should carry earplugs at all times to have them available whenever there is the realistic concern that sound will be uncomfortable. Being prepared to wear ear protection in those situations would not be considered a manifestation of phonophobia. It is actually a sensible fear that should motivate a person to always be prepared for the possibility of being exposed to sound that is uncomfortable.

If the precautions become extreme and persistent, then the person is doing more than what is necessary to protect against uncomfortable sound. Such *excessive* ear protection or avoidance of sound would define phonophobia, which might be thought of as *fear of sound that exceeds any reasonable concerns to take precautions against sound that is likely to be uncomfortable for any reason.*

Conducting the Assessment

The Sound Hypersensitivity Interview (chapter 5) offers the response option "avoid" for the different activities that are listed in questions 5 and 6. It would be unusual (but not impossible) for phonophobia to be an isolated condition, as it would normally exist along with loudness hyperacusis, pain hyperacusis, misophonia, and noise sensitivity. However, how do we distinguish between people *sensibly* protecting their ears from sound they know will be bothersome versus *excessively* protecting their ears when there is almost no chance of being exposed to uncomfortable sound? Making that distinction may require detailed questioning:

- What kinds of sounds are bothersome?
- When do you experience bothersome sounds?
- How do you protect yourself from bothersome sounds?

- *When* do you protect yourself from bothersome sounds?
  - ▸ Only when the sounds are likely to occur?
  - ▸ At times when the sounds are *not likely to occur*?

These questions will be implicitly answered in the process of conducting the Sound Hypersensitivity Interview (chapter 5). The main concern is whether the person is protecting from or avoiding sound even at times when experiencing bothersome sound is not likely, i.e., when there is no threat or danger.[61] It's healthy to fear the onset of sound that is known to be uncomfortable. The fear becomes unhealthy when protective measures are taken in the absence of any imminent threat that sound will be uncomfortable.

What Causes Phonophobia?

Appendix I provides a fairly detailed answer to this question. More briefly, the cause of phonophobia may involve mechanisms underlying the development of any specific phobia.

A traumatic experience can result in a specific phobia toward whatever caused the trauma.[61] Fear becomes associated with the event, and this *conditioned fear* can last a lifetime. Phobias can also develop without being associated with any experience. For example, fear of darkness is experienced by many children. The fear normally resolves, but it can become a specific phobia if "fear circuits" in the brain are dysfunctional.[61,65,66]

Traumatic noise (firecracker, airhorn blast, gunshot, etc.) and acoustic shock (see appendix E) can result in phonophobia due to the emotional impact of the traumatic event.[67-71] Phonophobia can also develop gradually without being associated with any event—normally because of the ongoing experience of loudness hyperacusis, pain hyperacusis, misophonia, or noise sensitivity. These disorders may develop during childhood. Misophonia often begins during childhood or early adolescence.[45]

Summary

Phonophobia has had inconsistent definitions as a type of sound hypersensitivity disorder. In the migraine literature, it refers to what would actually be loudness hyperacusis or noise sensitivity. Sometimes it refers to emotional reactions to sound, which would not normally be phobia-related. The key features of phonophobia are that it is an actual phobia and the main problem lies in the person's excessive fear that sound will cause discomfort, pain, and/or distress.

When diagnosing sound hypersensitivity disorders, it is most helpful to consider loudness hyperacusis and pain hyperacusis as disorders of physical discomfort. The physical discomfort can lead to emotional reactions, which would not be considered phonophobia—but could *lead* to phonophobia. Misophonia and noise sensitivity are by definition emotional disorders, and they also can lead to phonophobia. Phonophobia is a unique emotional disorder.

PART 4

Treating Sound Hypersensitivity Disorders

CHAPTER 11

Treating Sound Hypersensitivity Disorders: Important Considerations

A challenge when summarizing what is in the scientific literature regarding treatments for sound hypersensitivity disorders is the inconsistent terminology and definitions that are used to describe the various disorders. In their book, *Hyperacusis and Disorders of Sound Intolerance*, the editors Drs. Marc Fagelson and David Baguley commented on these inconsistencies, "All this may seem daunting, and lead one to consider that the topic of decreased sound tolerance cannot sensibly be addressed at all."[72] (p. vii) They noted, however, the field of *pain* had been in a similar conundrum, but the development of new therapies created a foundation upon which to conduct well-designed clinical trials. Their book was an attempt to "take a first step on a similar journey." The book you're reading is another step on that journey.

In spite of the inconsistent terminology and definitions in peer-reviewed publications, the scientific literature supports five distinctly different manifestations of a sound hypersensitivity disorder. New information could, of course, change the current thinking regarding these disorders. In fact, such new information is expected because this is such a new and undeveloped field of study. Hopefully this book will serve as an impetus to further distinguish between the different disorders and bring some uniformity to the field.

Chapters 3 through 10 describe procedures for screening, evaluating, and diagnosing sound hypersensitivity disorders. The terminology and definitions used in those chapters carry over to chapters 12 through 16 that describe treatment methods for the different disorders.

It is essential to make an accurate diagnosis to ensure that treatment is appropriate for the specific disorder. Chapter 4 contains a section titled Identifying the Primary Disorder to Prioritize Treatment. It might be helpful to review that section—key points are summarized below.

- If the primary disorder is diagnosed as loudness hyperacusis or pain hyperacusis, the hyperacusis receives priority treatment. Any associated emotions are treated as secondary to the underlying hyperacusis.
- If the primary complaint is emotional distress caused by sound:
  - ▸ The distress may be due to loudness hyperacusis or pain hyperacusis. If so, then the hyperacusis is the root cause of the emotions and should be the primary focus of treatment. The emotional distress would be treated as a secondary disorder.

▶ If loudness hyperacusis and pain hyperacusis can be ruled out, then the complaint may be diagnosed as misophonia, noise sensitivity, and/or phonophobia. Treating the emotions is the focus.

Desensitization Using Sound

Treatment of sound hypersensitivity disorders most typically involves systematic desensitization, specifically by gradually increasing exposure to the sound, or sounds, that are the source of discomfort. Whereas some practitioners recommend actually being forced to tolerate sounds that are uncomfortable, others recommend always keeping sound at a comfortable level. There may be no evidence to support one approach over the other, but my opinion is that desensitization procedures should not involve sounds that are annoying or uncomfortable in any way.

Counseling

Different forms of counseling are also commonly used as treatment for sound hypersensitivity disorders. The counseling may be mostly educational to provide information intended to dispel any fears about the disorder. Sometimes such education for *demystification* along with recommendations for how to self-administer sound desensitization are all that is needed. Structured methods of counseling include cognitive behavioral therapy (CBT), acceptance and commitment therapy, and mindfulness-based stress reduction. All of these methods can be helpful, and there is no evidence any one method is more effective than any other.

Whereas sound desensitization procedures are used to reduce auditory gain (appendix F), counseling techniques are primarily intended to reduce any negative emotions caused by a sound hypersensitivity disorder. In the next chapter we will review studies of CBT used to treat loudness hyperacusis. Those studies have generally shown success in reducing the emotional and social effects of the disorder. With any study, it is important to know which sound hypersensitivity disorder was treated, what treatment approach was used, and results of the treatment. That information is often not clear.

Determining the Appropriate Method of Treatment

Sound hypersensitivity disorders are distinctly different, and treatment should be appropriate to the particular disorder. Each of the five sound hypersensitivity disorders is listed below along with the approach to treatment that usually would be appropriate.

With *loudness hyperacusis*, the objective of treatment is to increase the person's tolerance to the loudness of everyday sounds. This is generally accomplished with a program of gradual desensitization using sound. Emotional reactions would be a secondary concern.

With *pain hyperacusis*, desensitization using sound may not be appropriate because *any* sound might be painful. The main objective for these people is to help them recover as normal a life as possible. This generally includes making lifestyle changes to quiet the environment. Counseling might be essential to help the person cope with the disorder. Sound therapy should be considered a possibility for the future but only if and when the person is ready.

Misophonia is an emotional disorder, so treatment should focus on reducing the emotional reactions caused by specific sounds. Depending on the individual's situation, treatment should involve counseling and/or a custom-tailored program of desensitization using sound.

Noise sensitivity is characterized by emotional reactions to sound in general. The sound hypersensitivity for these individuals is often linked to an emotional or psychological disorder. Treatment should address the root causes of the emotional reactions.

A person with *phonophobia* can have physical and/or emotional reactions to sound. Regardless of why sound hypersensitivity is a problem for the person, the reactions need to be reduced with appropriate treatment. The excessive fear, which defines phonophobia, should be addressed with appropriate counseling.

The specific treatment appropriate for an individual may be based on how the following questions are answered following the assessment:

1. Is the sound hypersensitivity disorder secondary to head injury?
2. What other health conditions are present? Hearing loss and use of hearing aids? Tinnitus? Anxiety, depression, PTSD, autism spectrum disorder? Symptoms of migraine?

3. Is the disorder thought to involve primarily the central auditory pathways, or are emotional and stress reactions the primary concern?
4. Does sound cause burning, stabbing, jabbing pain?
5. How much does the disorder impact the person's life?
6. Should an interdisciplinary approach be recommended? Can an audiologist provide the treatment, or should a psychologist or other psychological health provider be involved?
7. Is overprotection with earplugs and/or earmuffs a concern?
8. Is a fear response involved? Is the fear more of a reasonable concern or is it excessive?

Intensity of Treatment According to Level of Need

As part of the assessment, it is essential to determine whether a sound hypersensitivity disorder is mild, moderate, severe, or extreme with respect to its functional and emotional effects on the person. These different "degrees of life impact" are defined in chapter 4, starting with a *mild* disorder defined as "minimal but significant interference with normal life activities." If a loudness tolerance disorder is mild or even moderate, minimal counseling may be sufficient to alleviate any fears and to teach the person how to self-administer a sound therapy program of systematic desensitization without having to pay for expensive treatment or purchase special devices. If the disorder is severe, treatment should be rigorous and collaborative between clinician (audiologist and/or psychological health provider) and patient. Greater severity of the disorder might also warrant the purchase and use of special ear-level devices.

All of the treatments described in the upcoming chapters adhere to the principle of minimal treatment for a mild disorder and more intense treatment as necessary depending on the degree of impact caused by the disorder. Many people with a sound hypersensitivity disorder also have tinnitus. Sound desensitization procedures recommended for mild to moderate disorders can also be beneficial as sound therapy for reducing effects of tinnitus. Sound therapy can do double duty for these people, and often all the person needs is education to know how to self-administer sound therapy.

CHAPTER 12

Treating Loudness Hyperacusis

Appendix J addresses this question by summarizing studies that have been conducted to evaluate different methods of treatment for loudness hyperacusis. Based on those studies, we can suggest approaches to treatment that have research support. First, we'll briefly review the studies described in appendix J.

Two review articles are summarized in appendix J. The first was published in 2017 and involved a review of 43 studies, of which 19 specifically included treatment for hyperacusis.[24] Hyperacusis was defined in the review as "the perception of everyday environmental sound as being overwhelmingly loud or intense." [p. 1] Tinnitus Retraining Therapy (TRT) was the most commonly used treatment and was reported to be beneficial for most patients. Numerous limitations, however, led the authors to conclude, "There is a lack of sufficient evidence to identify effective management strategies." (p. 19)

The second review article was published in 2024 with a focus on sound therapy approaches of treatment for hyperacusis.[73] Hyperacusis was defined in the review using the consensus definition published in 2021:[16] "A reduced tolerance to sound(s) that are perceived as normal to the majority of the population or were perceived as normal to the person before their onset of hyperacusis." (p. 607) It was noted in chapter 3 that this consensus definition could apply to all sound hypersensitivity disorders—loudness hyperacusis, pain hyperacusis, misophonia, and noise sensitivity.

The authors of the 2024 review identified 31 studies that met their inclusion criteria.[73] Of the 31 studies, 23 reported using TRT. The other studies employed a variety of methods for using therapeutic sound. The authors concluded, "There is limited evidence supporting the use of sound therapy for patients with hyperacusis." (p. 10)

In addition to the two review articles, appendix J includes two reviews of studies that have evaluated the use of sound therapies for tinnitus. The first of these reviews combined hyperacusis with tinnitus and thus any conclusions could not be made about loudness hyperacusis specifically.[74] The second review also addressed both hyperacusis and tinnitus, with a focus on finding evidence for increased central auditory gain (appendix F) as the underlying mechanism.[75] They concluded the central auditory gain model has support in the literature and that both tinnitus and hyperacusis "conceivably should be effectively managed with sound therapy."

Finally, appendix J summarizes individual studies that evaluated different methods of treatment for hyperacusis (with varying definitions of hyperacusis). The methods evaluated included TRT, CBT, CBT combined with sound therapy, group education, "transitional intervention," and even surgery. Each of these methods has been shown to be of benefit to some people.

The studies summarized in appendix J reveal that the scientific literature does not provide definitive evidence regarding treatment methods for loudness hyperacusis. One of the problems is, of course, the lack of consistent terminology and definitions, which makes it difficult to comparatively evaluate the studies. This chapter takes these concerns into consideration when generalizing about viable methods of treatment that should be expected to benefit people with a loudness hyperacusis disorder.

Central Auditory Gain

To understand the rationale for why sound is used to desensitize the auditory system, it is important to understand the concept of *central auditory gain*, which is widely thought to be the mechanism most responsible for loudness hyperacusis.[19,35,68] One group refers to "hypergain neural activity within the central auditory pathways (the presumptive mechanism for loudness hyperacusis)."[76]

Appendix F provides a brief description of central auditory gain. I have also written about auditory gain in some detail in a previous book[26] (appendix A) and in a peer-reviewed publication.[77] In a nutshell, central auditory gain is thought to work like a volume control for sound that enters the ear. The volume (gain) is turned up for softer sounds and turned down for louder sounds. Central auditory gain is an essential human function because of the enormous range in sound intensity levels (as great as a 1,000,000,000,000-fold change) between the threshold of hearing and the level of loudness discomfort.[78] For the person with loudness hyperacusis, the upper end of this range is reduced to lower-than-normal levels. Treatment should have the effect of raising the upper end of this range to normal or close-to-normal levels. That treatment generally involves some type of systematic sound exposure to desensitize (or "recalibrate") central auditory gain.

Educational Counseling

The basic assumption of treatment for loudness hyperacusis is that heightened central auditory gain is the underlying cause of the disorder and sound therapy is the primary means of reducing the hypergain.[78] "To be successful, the patient must trust the clinician, who is essentially recommending an intervention that patients fear and that they may see as the opposite from their needs (i.e., increasing sound not decreasing it)."[79] (p. 228)

The relationship between sound and auditory gain must be understood to appreciate the rationale for using sound therapy as treatment to reset auditory gain to a lower level so that sound is not amplified as much. This relationship also explains why avoiding sound and overprotecting the ears with earplugs/earmuffs can reset auditory gain to a *higher* level and worsen the problem.

A study was conducted that perfectly depicts the relationship between sound and auditory gain.[33] Referring to this study is ideal for use as an educational tool to explain the relationship. The study is described in appendix F. Briefly, one group of participants wore ear-level sound generators for two weeks (*added-sound* group), and the second group wore earplugs for two weeks (*deprived-sound* group). The added-sound group experienced greater tolerance of the loudness of sounds, as demonstrated by an increase in their loudness discomfort levels (LDLs—see appendix A). The deprived-sound group experienced *reduced* loudness tolerance, as demonstrated by *decreased* LDLs. Results of this study, and of similar studies,[74,75,80] suggest that treatment of loudness hyperacusis should include both desensitization with sound therapy and appropriate use of hearing protection that avoids overprotection.

Educational counseling is intended to foster understanding and compliance with a sound desensitization protocol for which treatment focuses primarily on reducing the sensitivity of the auditory pathways. This type of counseling is not the same as counseling intended to reduce stress and emotional reactions that may accompany loudness hyperacusis. We will discuss that type of counseling later in this chapter.

Sound Therapy for Desensitization

Most of the methods for treating loudness hyperacusis have involved the use of sound in some manner to desensitize the central auditory pathways. The most common method is

TRT, which uses a specific form of sound therapy along with a structured counseling protocol.[24,73] Other methods that use different versions of sound therapy and counseling are Hyperacusis Activities Treatment (HAT) and Progressive Tinnitus Management (PTM). Transitional Intervention is a unique and relatively new approach for combining sound therapy with counseling to treat loudness hyperacusis. We'll discuss each of these methods below.

Tinnitus Retraining Therapy (TRT)

Patients evaluated for TRT are assigned to one of five treatment categories: 0, 1, 2, 3, or 4. Categories 0, 1, and 2 are specific to tinnitus.[27,81] For category 3 patients, sound hypersensitivity is the primary complaint, and the person may or may not have bothersome tinnitus.[82] Category 4 patients have prolonged worsening (exacerbation) of their tinnitus and/or their hyperacusis—caused by exposure to certain sounds. If loudness hyperacusis is the primary complaint for category 4 patients, then the treatment is the same as for category 3 patients.

The TRT category 3 protocol for treating loudness hyperacusis involves a modified version of the tinnitus counseling along with the use of ear-level sound generators.[27,81] If hearing difficulties are a significant problem for the person, then hearing aids with a built-in sound generator (combination instruments) are used. A less-severe loudness hyperacusis disorder might only require counseling, which would include suggestions for self-administered sound therapy.

The TRT counseling is oriented around the *neurophysiological model*, which describes three major areas of the brain.[27,81] The *auditory nervous system* processes sound; the *limbic system* processes emotions; the *autonomic nervous system* underlies stress and the fight-or-flight response. According to the model, loudness hyperacusis is defined by abnormally strong reactions (hypersensitivity) to sound within the auditory nervous system. Any sounds reaching a certain intensity level would consistently cause these reactions, which may activate the limbic and autonomic nervous systems. The primary objective of treatment is to reverse the hypersensitivity by *desensitizing* the auditory nervous system to sound—by decreasing the gain, or "turning down the volume." This is accomplished by systematic exposure to sounds that cause no annoyance or discomfort, which should result in a gradual increase in the ability to tolerate progressively louder sounds. With TRT, loudness discomfort levels (LDLs) are measured (see appendix A). If the desensitization procedure is successful, LDLs will increase in accordance with increased tolerance to the loudness of sounds. An increase in loudness tolerance may be observed in as little as a few weeks.

The originators of TRT claimed, "In most patients with the proper treatment, their problem with hyperacusis is resolved in half a year."[83] (p. 599) The review article mentioned at the beginning of this chapter and in appendix J commented, "The most commonly reported management strategy was TRT, and most studies indicated that the treatment was beneficial to patients with hyperacusis."[24]

Hyperacusis Activities Treatment (HAT)

The method of HAT is modeled after Tinnitus Activities Treatment.[84,85] HAT uses a combination of picture-based counseling and sound therapy. Depending on the person's specific problems, the counseling addresses thoughts and emotions, hearing and communication, sleep, and concentration. It is emphasized that, while earplugs or earmuffs are important when exposed to loud noise, the overuse of hearing protection can worsen hyperacusis. Custom-fit musician (high-fidelity) earplugs are recommended for "comfort in noisy situations."

Sound therapy with HAT can include low-level broadband noise to reduce central auditory gain or increasing the level of pleasant sounds (music, nature sounds, etc.) gradually over time.[84] For people with hearing loss requiring amplification, hearing aids can be adjusted to not amplify above the level that causes discomfort, with the *maximum power output* increased gradually over time. Hearing aids can even be used for people who don't have hearing loss. The hearing aids can initially function as earplugs to maintain comfort with all sounds. The maximum power output can be increased gradually, just as for people with hearing loss.

The HAT authors concluded, "Although there are currently no cures available for hyperacusis, there are several treatment options that can be successful for patients, including counseling, sound therapy, filtered earplugs, medications for related symptoms, and relaxation exercises."[84] (p. 172)

Progressive Tinnitus Management (PTM)

The treatment protocol for loudness hyperacusis with PTM was adapted from the approach used with TRT.[30,81] Both methods use a combination of sound therapy and counseling. The treatment protocol for TRT is described above.

With PTM, the intensity of treatment for a loudness hyperacusis disorder depends on the degree to which the disorder affects the person. In chapter 4 the different degrees (mild, moderate, severe, extreme) are defined. *Mild* loudness hyperacusis would receive minimal counseling and recommendations for using sound to desensitize the auditory system. *Moderate* loudness hyperacusis can be treated more intensely or less intensely, depending on the circumstances and the clinician's judgment as to what would best serve the person's needs.

Severe or extreme loudness hyperacusis would require intensive treatment, involving repeated counseling appointments and optimized sound therapy. The sound therapy might be most effective if ear-level devices are used (either wearable sound generators or combination instruments) to provide the greatest possible control over the therapeutic sound. If the person is being treated for bothersome tinnitus, the tinnitus treatment is suspended until the loudness hyperacusis is sufficiently resolved.

Regardless of the degree of the disorder's impact, treatment should include being in an environment of low-level background sound 24/7 for desensitization purposes. For people with bothersome tinnitus, the sound therapy can be helpful for both the loudness hyperacusis and the tinnitus problem.

The PTM flip-chart counseling guide contains a section that is specific to treating loudness hyperacusis.[86] Using this guide ensures that all of the essential counseling points are covered during the appointment.

Transitional Intervention

Transitional Intervention is described in some detail in appendix J. The method was published in a series of four "companion" reports.[76,78,87,88] Those reports provide considerable detail regarding the protocol.

The assumption is that people with loudness hyperacusis use avoidance behaviors, including the use of earplugs/earmuffs, to protect themselves from uncomfortably loud sound. These behaviors tend to sensitize the auditory system, which increases auditory gain (appendix F) and worsens the problem. The goal of Transitional Intervention is for people "to transition from their typical very quiet environment to a therapeutic sound-enriched environment and ultimately to routine sound environments and commonly experienced public places."[76] (p. 1869)

The use of therapeutic sound with "protective treatment devices" is the primary component of treatment. "The treatment motivation for sound therapy with bilateral sound generators is straightforward. The underlying assumption is that the mechanism that gives rise to loudness hyperacusis is maladaptive (abnormally increased) neural activity within the central auditory pathways. This hypergain process can be recalibrated (i.e., downregulated) and reset through use of controlled healthy sound exposure with the goals of reestablishing normal perception of loudness and typical sound tolerance."[76] (p. 1869)

The ear-level protective treatment devices were specially developed to protect the ears from uncomfortable sound and to gradually deliver increasing levels of broadband sound (and amplification) to the ears.[76] The structured counseling is essential to explain the rationale for sound therapy and how to optimize use of the protective treatment devices.[87] "Those familiar with TRT theory, the associated treatment principles, and the treatment model for hyperacusis should be at ease with this counseling approach."[88] (p. 1925)

At the time of this writing, Transitional Intervention is a new treatment. It has been patented through the US patent office and has been shown to be effective in a proof-of-concept trial.[88] The authors "plan to offer a counseling package, including a fully scripted protocol and a topical checklist together with a companion set of visual aids and diagrams. We also will include a list of selected publications that provide theoretical and clinical background for the counseling protocol and the protective management and sound treatment strategies that are the foundational components of our transitional intervention." (p. 1925)

Sound Therapy Apps

Sound therapy apps for smartphones are widely available on the internet. They are often advertised for meditation, relaxation, stress relief, and improving sleep. There are even hundreds of sound therapy apps specific to tinnitus.[89] Although few claim to be useful for loudness hyperacusis, most of them actually can be used as sound therapy for desensitization purposes.

Smartphones have numerous options for delivering sound to the ears. Many types of earbuds and earphones are available, including wireless devices. Special earbuds are available that allow for sound therapy during sleep. Most newer hearing aids have streaming capability, which enables sound therapy apps to deliver their signals wirelessly to the hearing aids. The sounds can be added to the amplification. The main concern is limiting the output of both the amplification and the sound therapy to ensure that sound is never uncomfortably loud.

All of the sound desensitization methods described in this chapter could conceivably use a sound therapy app. It might be argued that a constant level of broadband sound is optimal for desensitization purposes. It could also be argued that a variety of sounds could be used, as long as the sound enrichment is continuous. Research has not shown any particular type of sound or schedule of sound therapy to be optimal. It seems likely that sound therapy, regardless of the source and the delivery system, should be constant throughout both the day and night.

Cognitive Behavioral Therapy (CBT)

CBT is a psychological intervention that has been shown to be effective for treating pain, anxiety, depression, and insomnia.[90] CBT was adapted for treatment of tinnitus and has considerable research evidence for this purpose.[91-93] Importantly, CBT treats the *effects* of tinnitus (disrupted sleep, concentration difficulties, emotional reactions), not the *sensation* of tinnitus (the sound itself).

Similarly, CBT can be used to treat emotional reactions to loudness hyperacusis but not the underlying auditory gain—at least not directly. CBT has been used to treat *sound-avoidance behaviors* that are associated with loudness hyperacusis.[94] By reducing sound avoidance, more sound enters the ears, which helps desensitize the auditory system (an indirect form of sound therapy). Thus, CBT can be used to reduce both anxiety associated with loudness hyperacusis and sound-avoidance behaviors.

Appendix J reviews studies of CBT for hyperacusis, with generally favorable outcomes. If a person has anxiety or other negative emotions caused by loudness hyperacusis, then CBT would be appropriate to treat the emotions. Treating sound-avoidance behaviors can also be helpful to increase exposure to sound for desensitization purposes.

CBT Combined with Sound Therapy

CBT can be offered as a "counseling-only" strategy for treating loudness hyperacusis. Generally, it would be expected that CBT offered with some form of sound therapy would be optimal. Two studies support this supposition, which are summarized in appendix J.[95,96]

Recommendation for CBT

In summary, the use of CBT to treat loudness hyperacusis should include counseling to reduce sound-avoidance behaviors, some form of appropriate sound therapy, and counseling to reduce any emotional reactions—generally involving anxiety, depression, irritation, frustration, and anger.

Migraine-Based Treatment

The association between migraine and inner ear disorders, including loudness hyperacusis, is described in appendix E.

Appendix J describes a trial to evaluate "multi-modal pro-phylaxis therapy" as treatment for hyperacusis that resulted in the majority of patients experiencing "symptomatic improvement."[97] The treatment is referred to as "multi-modal" because it involves a combination of treatments, including lifestyle and dietary changes, medications, and targeted nutraceuticals (food-derived substances with purported medical benefits) directed to *atypical migraine* (symptoms of migraine without severe headaches). The treatment is *prophylactic* as *prevention* of atypical migraine, which is thought to cause hyperacusis by the authors of the trial, and more effective than traditional treatments used for migraine headaches.

Treatment was described as follows: "patients were counseled on implementing lifestyle modifications. This included dietary modifications, which consisted of avoiding foods containing certain preservatives, fermented prod-ucts, chocolate, nuts, eggs, alcohol, fresh breads/yeast products, aged/processed meats, certain beans, certain fruit (high histamine), and pickled or preserved fruit/ vegetables. In addition, dietary supplementation with mag-nesium 400 mg bid [twice a day] riboflavin (vitamin B2) 200 mg bid was prescribed. We did not restrict sodium intake as long as the patient stayed well-hydrated. Patients were also instructed to eat three meals and sleep on a regular schedule on weekends and weekdays to avoid fatigue, hunger, and dehydration. The patients were also prescribed pharmacologic migraine prophylaxis in a step-wise agent- and dose-escalating manner."[97] [(p. 3)] Please see the article (which is open-access) for details of the drug regimen.

Hamid Djalilian, MD and his research group have conducted years of research, and he writes (personal communication): "Hyperacusis is related to a migraine-related central sensitivity syndrome. Traditionally, migraine has been thought to be a headache disorder. In recent years, migraine has been found to be associated with many other non-headache disorders. This atypical form of migraine often causes ear symptoms, termed *otologic migraine.* Otologic migraine patients may experience symptoms such as hyperacusis, increased tinnitus loudness, vertigo and dizziness, sudden hearing loss, motion sickness, among others. These patients may have neck stiffness, sinus pain/pressure, aural pressure or pain, and may not ever have experienced a headache. Atypical migraine (non-headache migraine) causes sensitivity at the brain level, which causes central amplification of the peripheral signal and leads to hyperacusis. The same increased central sensitivity enhances the perception of tinnitus. The atypical migraine phenomenon is likely what links tinnitus and hyperacusis in many patients. A comprehensive treatment approach to atypical migraine can reduce the central sensitivity, and hence reduce the hypersensitivity to sound and the loudness of tinnitus."

Loudness Hyperacusis Associated with Autism Spectrum Disorders

Loudness hyperacusis is highly prevalent in people with autism spectrum disorders, as reviewed in appendix E. Treating the autistic population can involve any of the treatments described in this chapter. Importantly, the symptoms may define noise sensitivity or misophonia, rather than loudness hyperacusis, hence the need for an accurate diagnosis.

Often, autistic children require treatment for sound hypersensitivity. They may overuse hearing protection, which provides a sense of safety but can exacerbate the problem—as mentioned often in this book. For this population, reducing the use of ear protection and providing sound therapy "should be done with more tact and in a more gradual timeline."[98] (p. 551) Sound therapy should include both enriching the environment with pleasant sounds and desensitization training to undesirable sounds. Sounds that are bothersome to the person can be downloaded for playback, starting at very low levels and gradually increasing the volume weekly.

No studies to date have reported on the use of CBT to treat loudness hyperacusis in the autistic population.[98] It has been shown, however, that they respond well to CBT aimed at reducing anxiety, which can be a major concern with sound hypersensitivity. Another treatment that has been used is auditory integration training, but it "has little credible data demonstrating its effectiveness." (p. 554)

Loudness Hyperacusis Associated with Brain Injury

As noted in appendix E, traumatic brain injury (TBI) can have so many symptoms that a multidisciplinary approach to treatment is necessary.[99] Further, loudness hyperacusis

associated with TBI cannot be assumed to be a central auditory gain problem. A TBI can damage any component of the
auditory system—from the eardrum to the auditory cortex.
Treatment for sound hypersensitivity associated with TBI
therefore may require a different approach. The treatment
may consist of approaches that are used to treat auditory
processing disorder, such as auditory training (to "sharpen
specific auditory functions"), assistive devices for hearing
(such as an ear-level frequency modulation [FM] system),
and communication counseling.[99]

Surgery

Surgery might be a last resort, but there is evidence for
a surgical technique that has been used to treat loudness
hyperacusis.[100] The technique is summarized in appendix
J. In essence, "minimally invasive" middle ear surgery
impedes the transmission of sound waves to the cochlea,
which effectively reduces the loudness of sound. The
majority of patients undergoing this procedure showed
improvement in hyperacusis symptoms, which was sustained for an average of two years following the surgery.

Summary

Loudness hyperacusis is widely believed to be a disorder
normally caused by heightened central auditory gain
(appendix F). Different forms of sound therapy have been
developed for purposes of decreasing the gain. There is

considerable evidence that this approach is often effective (appendix J). The optimal method of sound therapy, however, is undetermined. "Sound therapy is not a cure, but done properly it helps, potentially a lot, I'm convinced of that." (Dr. Martin Pienkowski, personal communication)

An audiologist can provide sound therapy to reduce auditory gain, and a psychologist or other psychological healthcare provider can treat any associated emotional reactions or insomnia. Treatment of loudness hyperacusis thus often requires an interdisciplinary team approach. Although controversial, studies have shown that audiologists can deliver CBT to treat both tinnitus and hyperacusis.[101-103]

If treatment successfully resolves the physical discomfort caused by sound, then the cause of any associated emotional reactions would be eliminated. This assumption might be used as an argument to just treat the physical symptoms while ignoring any associated emotional distress or insomnia. That argument would be mistaken, however, because an indeterminate amount of time is needed to treat the physical symptoms, with no guarantee they will be resolved. Ignoring the negative emotions would not be appropriate—nor ethical. Any emotional reactions and/or insomnia should be treated simultaneously with the sound desensitization procedures.

Finally, loudness hyperacusis can have a cause unrelated to auditory gain. We've discussed loudness hyperacusis associated with migraine, autism spectrum disorders, and brain injury—all of which can have different mechanisms underlying the sound hypersensitivity disorder. If sound therapy is not effective, then other types of treatment should be considered. In all cases, educational counseling is essential so that patients understand why the treatment is expected to be beneficial. Counseling for emotional reactions is also essential, which may be done in conjunction with any treatment targeted to the underlying physical disorder.

CHAPTER 13

Treating Pain Hyperacusis

Pain hyperacusis is also referred to as *noxacusis* (see appendix G).[39] The disorder is not understood by the majority of healthcare professionals.[37] "In desperation for support and medical advice, many individuals with pain hyperacusis seek counsel on social media. Avoiding healthcare professionals and seeking counsel from non-medical sources complicates the ability to take a structured approach to treatment."[37 (p. 18)]

For this chapter, there are few sources to draw from to describe available treatments for pain hyperacusis. Those sources, however, are rich with insights about the disorder and what types of treatment approaches may be options.

Sound Therapy

We discussed in the previous chapter how sound therapy is the go-to method of treatment for loudness hyperacusis. The underlying premise is that loudness hyperacusis is caused by abnormally heightened auditory gain (appendix F), and that systematic stimulation with sound can reduce (desensitize) the auditory gain, resulting in the ability to tolerate higher levels of sound.[78] That premise is not an assumption for pain hyperacusis. Different possible mechanisms underlying pain hyperacusis are described in appendix G and do not include heightened auditory gain.

It has been reported that sound therapy worsened pain hyperacusis for some patients.[3,5,37] These studies, however, found that many of these individuals were "self-administering" sound therapy because they do not trust healthcare professionals. One individual with pain hyperacusis reported that sound therapy was "counterproductive and lowered my sound tolerance dramatically. I never recovered from that worsening."[6] (p. 31)

It is clear that sound therapy can be ineffective for some people with pain hyperacusis and can even worsen the disorder. There are, however, some people who seem to benefit from sound therapy. What is unknown is whether those who benefit have pain hyperacusis that is not associated with enhanced auditory gain.

For a person diagnosed with pain hyperacusis, it is important to understand these concerns with sound therapy. If sound causes any degree of discomfort, then sound therapy is not an option. However, *sound therapy should not be ruled out as future treatment* depending on the person's ability to start tolerating sound. Other methods of treatment may improve the person's condition such that some sound can be tolerated. At that point, sound can be introduced at a low level and very gradually and systematically increased over time. Regardless of the underlying mechanism, successful treatment requires that the auditory system become tolerant of sound. A program of sound therapy should therefore be implemented if at all possible. It would be essential that any sound used for therapy is comfortably tolerated and never annoying, uncomfortable, or painful.

Pharmaceutical and Non-Pharmaceutical Treatments Reported by Jahn et al. (2025)

Perhaps the best source of data on different treatments used for pain hyperacusis is a study by Dr. Kelly Jahn and colleagues.[37] In this study, 32 adults with pain hyperacusis described their use of pharmaceutical and non-pharmaceutical treatments for pain relief. "The present study shows that individuals with pain hyperacusis try many different types of pharmaceutical and non-pharmaceutical interventions that are often self-prescribed. This unstructured treatment approach makes it difficult to identify the treatments and doses that provide pain relief." [pp. 18-19] Considering this limitation, we can look at the wide variety of treatments that were reported along with their perceived effectiveness, which was rated as follows:

- Excellent effect (>90% pain relief)
- Modest effect (>75% pain relief)
- Somewhat effective (50% pain relief)
- No effect (0% pain relief)
- Made my noxacusis worse

Pharmaceutical Treatments

Two of the participants used *opioid medications* (widely used for all types of pain, but associated with serious risks). One reported an "excellent effect" using oxycodone. The other reported that tramadol was "somewhat effective."

Non-opioid medications were used by 17 of the participants with mixed results. *Benzodiazepines* (which depress the central nervous system to produce a calming effect; examples: clonazepam, alprazolam) were used by 10 participants. Of these, one reported an "excellent effect"; two reported a "modest effect"; two reported they were "somewhat effective"; four reported "no effect"; and one reported "made my noxacusis worse."

Antidepressants (used to relieve symptoms of depression; examples: amitriptyline, clomipramine, duloxetine) were used by nine participants. Of these, two said they were "somewhat effective" and seven said they had "no effect."

NSAIDs (*non-steroidal anti-inflammatory drugs* used to reduce pain, fever, and inflammation; examples: ibuprofen, naproxen) were used by eight participants. Of these, five said they were "somewhat effective" and three said they had "no effect."

Muscle relaxants (reduce tension in muscles; used to treat cerebral palsy, multiple sclerosis, stroke, tension headache, low back pain, and fibromyalgia; examples: baclofen, cyclobenzaprine) were used by six participants. Four said they were "somewhat effective" and two said they had "no effect."

Anticonvulsants (help control nerve impulses; used to treat seizure disorders and epilepsy; examples: gabapentin, pregabalin, carbamazepine) were used by six participants. One reported an "excellent effect" and one reported a "modest effect." Two said they were "somewhat effective" and two said they had "no effect."

Nerve blockers (block pain signaling in nerves; examples: lidocaine, ambroxol) were used by four participants. Two reported an "excellent effect" and two reported "no effect."

Botox (neurotoxin—*botulinum toxin*—that temporarily paralyzes muscles; injected into the tensor veli palatini muscle to prevent it from contracting—see Middle Ear Muscle Disorders in appendix E) was used by one participant who reported "excellent effect."

Other medications included *Tylenol* (pain reliever and fever reducer; used by two participants—one reported a "modest effect" and the other reported "somewhat effective"), *flunarizine* (used for many purposes such as preventing migraine and vertigo; used by one participant—"no effect"), and *valacyclovir* (antiviral medication used to treat shingles; used by one participant—"somewhat effective").

Finally, cannabinoids (marijuana, THC, and/or CBD) were used by 10 participants.[37] Nine reported "no effect" and one reported "made my noxacusis worse."

"The perceived effectiveness of these pharmaceutical interventions varied. Out of the 63 effectiveness ratings provided across all pharmaceutical interventions, 56% of the ratings indicated that the treatment had no effect on pain hyperacusis and 3% indicated the treatment made their pain hyperacusis worse. Some patients reported modest-to-excellent effects from benzodiazepines, nerve blockers, anticonvulsants, Tylenol, oxycodone, and Botox.... Cannabinoids were consistently rated as ineffective for pain relief."[37] (pp. 13-14)

Non-Pharmaceutical Treatments

Non-pharmaceutical treatments were used by 20 of the 32 participants. *Meditation, yoga, or mindfulness therapy* was used by 12 participants with one of these reporting "somewhat effective" and 11 reporting "no effect." Similarly, *counseling* was used by 11 participants with one of these reporting "somewhat effective" and 10 reporting "no effect." *Cognitive behavioral therapy* was used by nine participants—one reported "excellent effect"; one reported "somewhat effective"; and seven reported "no effect."

Sound therapy was used by eight participants—one reported "excellent effect"; one reported "modest effect"; two reported "no effect"; and four reported "made my noxacusis worse." Tinnitus Retraining Therapy (TRT) was used by five participants—three reported "no effect" and two reported "made my noxacusis worse."

Two participants used *TMJ (temporomandibular joint) physical therapy*—one reported "excellent effect" and one reported "no effect." Two participants used *chiropractor or massage therapy*—one reported "modest effect" and one reported "somewhat effective."

A number of therapies were reported by one participant each: *round and oval window reinforcement* (see Surgery section in appendix J; "no effect"); *prism lens therapy* (normally used to treat binocular vision disorders; "modest effect"); *low-level laser therapy* (low-powered laser delivered to the eardrum; "modest effect"); *pranic energy healing* (prana, or life force energy, is used to restore balance in the body; "somewhat effective"); *TMJ splint therapy* (dental appliance molded to cover teeth; "excellent effect"); *dry needling* (insertion of needles to stimulate trigger points in muscles; "no effect"); *acupuncture* ("no effect"); and *prayer* ("no effect").

"Non-pharmaceutical interventions were largely ineffective at providing pain relief in our cohort. Out of the 57 efficacy ratings provided across all non-pharmaceutical interventions, most indicated that these treatments had no effect on pain hyperacusis or that these interventions made their noxacusis worse. All six participants who experienced a worsening of their noxacusis indicated that this occurred after therapies that involved a sound exposure component (i.e., sound therapy or tinnitus retraining therapy)."[37] (p. 14)

Other Treatments for Pain Hyperacusis

Myriam Westcott (2016)

This report focused on hyperacusis linked to tonic tensor tympani syndrome (appendixes E and G) caused by a lowering of the threshold for tensor tympani muscle activity.[104] Many symptoms can result from the frequent spasm (myoclonus) of the muscle. Symptoms related to pain hyperacusis would include sharp, stabbing ear pain, dull earache, sensation of ear blockage (aural fullness), and "pain/numbness/ burning around the ear."

"If patients are not given an explanation of their symptoms, the resultant anxiety and distress can play a role not only in tinnitus and hyperacusis escalation but also in limiting the degree of efficacy of therapeutic intervention. Explaining tonic tensor tympani syndrome provides validation, reassurance and helps reduce anxiety, which can have an immediate effect on reducing the symptoms." [(p. 1)]

To manage the pain, treatment includes medication for nerve pain, and exercises provided by a physiotherapist "to relax the facial muscles in and around the ear and guidance in locating muscle trigger points in the neck, shoulder and arm. Patients carrying out these exercises plus gentle self-massage of their trigger points report benefit in reducing the intensity of their pain and in managing flare-ups. Interestingly, in some hyperacusis patients, this can also reduce hyperacusis severity.... surgical cutting of the tensor tympani muscle is a last resort and in my experience generally only partly effective in symptom reduction." [(pp. 1-2)]

Noreña et al. (2018)

This group hypothesized that acoustic shocks and traumas (and "potentially also after other non-auditory causes") can result in a cluster of debilitating auditory symptoms, including hyperacusis, ear fullness and tension, and ear pain.[71] Their model proposes that injury of the tensor tympani muscle leads to inflammation, which activates the trigeminal nerve (appendix G) and its connections in the brain.

For treatment, they suggest "several clinical approaches may be used to improve a patient condition. One strategy involves incapacitating the tensor tympani muscle by severing it. This treatment has been used experimentally in Ménière's disease. This surgery results in an improvement in perception [hearing] thresholds, tinnitus, feeling of ear fullness, and vertigo.... Pharmacological approaches, such as the use of muscle relaxants or anticholinergic agents

(Botox), could also be considered to reduce tensor tympani muscle contractions…. Methods using analgesics or anti-inflammatory agents could be efficient. Moreover, muscle tone and pain being possibly under the modulation of the sympathetic nervous system, blocking the sympathetic nervous system may improve the symptom cluster…. An autonomic nerve blocker administered intravenously has been shown to reduce the sensation of aural fullness, which is possibly related to tensor tympani muscle contraction."[71] (p. 12)

The authors noted that emotions may modulate contractions of the tensor tympani muscle. "It is therefore probable that behavioral approaches for stress and anxiety reduction, such as relaxation or behavioral and cognitive therapies…. can affect tensor tympani muscle tonicity and triggering threshold. By promoting tensor tympani muscle relaxation, these methods could contribute to minimize or even abolish tonic tensor tympani syndrome symptoms."[71] (p. 12)

Williams et al. (2021)

This study analyzed differences between 91 people with loudness hyperacusis compared to 152 with pain hyperacusis.[3] Individuals who reported experiencing ear pain "every day" or "continuously" were classified as having pain hyperacusis. Those reporting pain weekly or less were classified as having loudness hyperacusis. The authors noted that their definition of pain hyperacusis was not consensual and that further research is needed to clearly distinguish between the loudness and pain subgroups.

Included in the comparison between groups was how individuals *responded to treatment*. Those with loudness hyperacusis reported more benefit from sound therapy than those with pain hyperacusis. "One notable finding was that individuals with loudness hyperacusis were more likely to report substantial improvement with sound therapy than individuals with pain hyperacusis, although approximately one third of pain hyperacusis patients reported at least minor improvement." (p. 354)

Three types of medications were reported to be of benefit. Thirty individuals reported benefit from benzodiazepines; eight from opioids; and ten from *gabapentinoids* (used to treat many disorders, including epilepsy, neuropathic pain, insomnia, migraine, and panic disorder).[3] "Gabapentinoids and opioids were both only reported as beneficial in patients with pain hyperacusis, indicating that certain medications targeting nociceptive symptoms may be specifically useful for individuals with pain hyperacusis but not loudness hyperacusis." (p. 354) The authors strongly cautioned "against the routine prescribing of benzodiazepines for patients with hyperacusis, although judicious use of these medications (with frequent re-assessment of benefits and harms) may be warranted in some cases." (p. 355)

The authors acknowledged that a limitation of their study was a lack of data "on the perceived efficacy of cognitive-behavioral therapy (CBT)." They noted, however, "Future research investigating the utility of CBT as a potential treatment for hyperacusis should specifically investigate the degree to which response to CBT may differ between individuals with and without pain hyperacusis. Notably, as CBT has demonstrated efficacy in treating other forms of chronic pain with diverse etiologies, the adaptation of existing CBT protocols to pain hyperacusis remains a potentially fruitful area of future research."[3] (p. 355)

Fournier et al. (2022)

This study was conducted "to provide further insights into the mechanisms of tonic tensor tympani syndrome."[105] (p. 2) (Tonic tensor tympani syndrome is described in appendix E.) They measured middle ear function in 11 patients who reported these symptoms. One of the patients reported results of his treatment for pain hyperacusis.

The patient was treated with *clonazepam* (a benzodiazepine sedative used to treat panic disorders and seizures). Some minor improvement was noted in his ability to tolerate louder sounds. That treatment was stopped, and Botox was injected into the tensor tympani and levator veli palatini muscles (see appendix E). A month later, the patient did not experience pain in the ear after being exposed to impulsive sound. "These results suggest that some muscle activity in the oro-facial area was responsible for the pain and was deactivated by the toxin." (p. 29)

Shelley Witt (2023)

Shelley Witt is an audiologist at the University of Iowa who treated loudness hyperacusis successfully with sound therapy until she had a patient with pain hyperacusis.[5] For that patient, sound therapy "quickly made the condition worse.... People with loudness hyperacusis are bothered and might even feel pain, but it is not debilitating. They don't have the same type of pain as individuals with pain hyperacusis, and they don't have setbacks."

This article concludes that it's wrong to advise patients with pain hyperacusis to stop wearing earplugs or earmuffs or to use sound therapy. The recommendation is for *lifestyle modifications*. "Most of these people are already doing modifications because it's the only way they can get through the day. Such modifications generally include soundproofing at home, giving up typical kitchen dishes in favor of paper plates, and wearing ear protection for dangers like food packaging, etc."

David Treworgy (2023)

David Treworgy (author of this book's Foreword) is an individual who had experienced pain hyperacusis for about 10 years prior to the publication of his article.[6] His journey to seek help started with a visit to a primary care physician and then to an otolaryngologist (ear, nose, and throat doctor—ENT). He was told by the ENT that there was no specific treatment but that supplements might help. He tried them and they were not helpful.

He then received treatment with Tinnitus Retraining Therapy (TRT). This involved wearing ear-level sound generators that provided low-level broadband noise that was increased in volume very slowly over months. The treatment "turned out to be counterproductive and lowered my sound tolerance dramatically."

A year later, he "underwent a surgical clinical trial for hyperacusis called round window reinforcement. This surgery [see appendix J] functions in some ways as a permanent earplug, building up a layer of tissue to dampen incoming sound. Though some patients reported improvement, unfortunately I was not one of them.... A year after surgery, as a shot in the dark, I tried a stem cell transplant, which did not help either, but at least it did not make things worse."

"Much of the advice available from clinicians and online about hyperacusis is that 'everyday sounds cannot hurt you'; that you must 'push your way through the pain' and 'live your life.' I followed this terrible advice at first and unfortunately I found my ears got much worse."

Summary

In spite of the numerous approaches that have been used to treat pain hyperacusis, it seems we are left with more questions than answers. Pain hyperacusis is a relatively unknown disorder, and a variety of theories attempt to explain the underlying mechanism responsible for causing the painful symptoms. Successful treatment depends on understanding the underlying mechanism.

In this chapter, pertinent information in the scientific literature has been summarized. Fortunately, the limited studies that are available provide valuable insights for treatment options. On the other hand, the literature provides no definitive guidance as to how to treat pain hyperacusis.

Sound therapy may not be an option for some people who have pain hyperacusis as defined in this book. As mentioned, however, it is important to leave the door open for possible sound therapy in the future, even if sound cannot be tolerated *at all* at the time of diagnosis. After all, the ultimate goal of therapy for pain hyperacusis is that the person is comfortable with reasonable levels of sound. Under no circumstances should the person be advised to "tough it out" by enduring painful sound under the pretense that sound exposure will eventually result in the ability to tolerate sound comfortably.

Counseling is essential for all people with pain hyperacusis. Educational counseling should be used to explain what is known about pain hyperacusis and possible treatments.[104] Counseling to reduce stress and anxiety should be done as needed, which may also have the benefit of relaxing the tensor tympani muscle.[71] Cognitive behavioral therapy (CBT) may not be supported by research studies, but its efficacy in treating other forms of pain suggests that CBT might be helpful and certainly would not cause any harm.[3]

Possibly the best source for treatment options is the study described above for pharmaceutical and non-pharmaceutical treatments.[37] In that study, "most participants reported low efficacy of interventions that are designed to counteract maladaptive gain in the central nervous system (e.g., sound therapy, tinnitus retraining therapy) and six participants reported that those therapies made their noxacusis worse."[37]

Two of the participants had an "excellent effect (>90% pain relief)" using nerve blockers (lidocaine and ambroxol).[37] Extensive evidence supports ambroxol for treating neuropathic pain in various conditions. One participant reported an excellent effect from Botox injections in the tensor veli palatini muscle (see appendix E). "The tensor veli palatini is innervated by the trigeminal motor root and may form a functional unit with the tensor tympani muscle to control middle ear pressure.... we feel that our results are most consistent with trigeminal nerve involvement. This hypothesis can be clinically tested in the future using locally administered analgesics such as over-the-counter 4% lidocaine ear drops, a common treatment for pain due to acute otitis media in young children."[37]

Results of this study showed modest-to-excellent effects from pharmaceutical treatment with benzodiazepines, nerve blockers, anticonvulsants, Tylenol, oxycodone, and Botox.[37] The non-pharmaceutical treatments were "largely ineffective."

Another study reviewed in this chapter showed promising results with benzodiazepines, opioids, and gabapentinoids—with a strong warning to use benzodiazepines "judiciously."[3] Another study noted some minor improvement with clonazepam.[105] The audiologist from the University of Iowa recommended lifestyle modifications.[5] David Treworgy was an example of a patient who tried many treatments without success.[6]

Results of these various studies do not provide solid evidence to recommend any specific treatment for pain hyperacusis. The first challenge is diagnosing the disorder. Not only is the distinction between pain hyperacusis and loudness hyperacusis unclear, but the two variations are often not even recognized as being separate disorders. Pain hyperacusis is indeed a distinct disorder with likely multiple variations. Clinicians need training to understand the potential underlying mechanisms to most accurately treat the source of the pain. Hopefully the information provided in this book will be helpful in contributing toward the development of consensus regarding these related disorders, how to diagnose them, and how to treat them.

CHAPTER 14

Treating Misophonia

Treatment of misophonia differs significantly from treating hyperacusis.[106] The main objective of treatment for *loudness* hyperacusis is to reduce the sensitivity of the auditory pathways (chapter 12). With *pain* hyperacusis, the objective is to alleviate the pain that results from exposure to low to moderate levels of sound (chapter 13). For misophonia, the primary objective is to reduce emotional reactions caused by "trigger sounds." Treatment of misophonia requires "extensive counseling and takes more time than the treatment of hyperacusis."[106] (p. 8)

"Although understanding of misophonia is increasing, there is a great deal that is unknown about the condition, and even less about its treatment."[107] (p. 2) Treating misophonia is particularly challenging for a number of reasons: (1) Affected individuals vary greatly with respect to the sounds that trigger their reactions as well as how they react to those sounds. (2) It seems likely there are different forms of misophonia that have yet to be identified. (3) It is not clear whether misophonia should be considered an auditory disorder or a psychological/psychiatric disorder. (4) Research-based treatments for misophonia are limited and most trials have focused on different versions of cognitive behavioral therapy (CBT).[107]

Complicating the question of how to most effectively treat misophonia is the lack of agreement regarding which medical discipline should manage the disorder. "The question 'Does misophonia belong to the field of otolaryngology, audiology, neurophysiology, neurology, psychology, or psychiatry?' is significant."[106] (p. 8) That question is indeed significant and also currently unanswerable. It is essential to inform clinicians in each of these disciplines about misophonia and to encourage them to take an interest in offering the needed clinical services. Coordination and collaboration between disciplines is the optimal approach to address this complex disorder.

Systematic Review of Treatments for Misophonia

A summary of treatments for misophonia can be found in a systematic review of misophonia treatments that was published in 2023.[108] This was a review of research "to examine the preliminary evidence for various treatment modalities.... the treatment had to specifically target misophonia symptoms." (pp. 2-3) Results of their review are summarized below.

Cognitive Behavioral Therapy

"Of all the treatment approaches studied to date, cognitive-behavioral therapy (CBT) is the most consistently effective."[108] (p. 4) Numerous studies have evaluated CBT for misophonia, of which only one was a randomized controlled trial. That trial enrolled 54 adult patients who were randomized to either receive weekly group therapy for three months or to be placed on a waiting list (no treatment).[109] For the CBT group, "effects were modest and maintained at 1-year follow-up, suggesting short and long term benefit for misophonia symptoms."[108] (p. 5) These results were consistent with a previous *open-label study* (both researchers and participants were aware of the treatment method) conducted by the same research group evaluating 90 patients who were treated for misophonia using a similar CBT approach.[110]

The randomized controlled trial for CBT involved a combination of psychotherapy and psychomotor therapy (a holistic approach that recognizes the strong connection between mind and body).[109] The authors concluded their trial "provides evidence for the efficacy of CBT for misophonia and can serve as a stepping stone to implement CBT in clinical practice. We have published our protocol, so more misophonia patients can benefit from this treatment." (p. 715)

A specific technique used in the randomized controlled trial was *counterconditioning*.[108] For treating misophonia, this technique involves pairing a positive auditory stimulus (such as music) with a negative trigger stimulus (such as chewing), while inducing relaxation (using progressive muscle relaxation, for example). Relaxation would normally be incompatible with the usual reactions that occur in response to a trigger—hence the name counterconditioning.

Multiple *case studies* (that report results from a single person) have shown both in-person and remote delivery of CBT to be beneficial for treating misophonia.[108] Different components of CBT were used in these studies, making it difficult to know which components were the most effective. Of note, the person's family can be included in the sessions, which may increase the overall benefit of therapy.

Some case studies used *exposure techniques* whereby people were exposed to trigger stimuli while in a safe environment.[108] Different forms of exposure therapy were used between the studies. Using exposure techniques generally required longer therapy and more intense sessions than CBT that did not include exposure therapy.

Tinnitus Retraining Therapy

The authors of this systematic review considered Tinnitus Retraining Therapy (TRT) to be a type of exposure therapy.[108] In a sense it is, but that aspect of the treatment needs to be understood within the full context of TRT (see chapter 12 and appendix J). It will be explained here how TRT is adapted to treat misophonia. We will then look at the studies of TRT used for misophonia that were reported in this systematic review.

The overall approach of TRT is to provide counseling that is based on the neurophysiological model along with a specific form of sound therapy.[27,81] Very briefly, the neurophysiological model consists of the auditory nervous system (which processes sound), the limbic system (which processes emotions), and the autonomic nervous system (which underlies stress and the fight-or-flight response).

The neurophysiological model provides the foundation for all of the counseling with TRT.

The treatment protocol with TRT has been adapted to treat hyperacusis (see chapter 12) and misophonia.[111] Both the counseling and the sound therapy differ substantially when treating hyperacusis versus misophonia. For hyperacusis, "counseling and sound therapy focus on mechanisms of general desensitization to sound provided by constant, 24/7 exposure to neutral sound, and the general enrichment of environmental sounds.... Our clinical experience shows that treatment which is effective for hyperacusis is not helpful for misophonia."[106] (p. 8)

To understand the rationale for how TRT is used to treat misophonia, it is important to understand the concept of *conditioned reflexes*.[27,112] Many of our daily activities do not require conscious attention—things like walking, driving a car, and brushing our teeth. These types of *automatic behaviors* become second nature—they can be performed with little or no conscious thought. They are the result of conditioned reflexes.

Misophonia "arises from the creation of subconscious functional connections governed by principles of conditioned reflexes."[106] (p. 8) These connections exist between the auditory, limbic, and autonomic nervous systems.[81] Misophonia "involves the same connections and mechanisms as tinnitus and is controlled by conditioned reflexes. Basically, all principles and explanations used for tinnitus are applicable for misophonia, with the difference that the neuronal activity evoked [triggered] by external sound acts in place of tinnitus-related neuronal activity. However, it is linked to the reactions of the limbic and autonomic nervous system in entirely the same fashion as clinically significant tinnitus. Therefore, the same basic approach of extinction of conditioned reflexes can be utilized for the treatment of misophonia."[81] (p. 107)

Sound therapy used for misophonia "focuses on creating a positive association to sound in general and on decreasing/removing negative reactions to misophonic triggers."[106] (p. 8) Creating positive associations with sound in general can be accomplished by *active listening* to pleasant sounds.[81,113] Active listening is contrasted with *passive* listening, which refers to sounds we can hear but don't pay attention to. When misophonia and hyperacusis occur together, sound therapy should involve both active listening to pleasant sounds to address the misophonia and desensitization of the auditory system to address the hyperacusis (which can be accomplished with passive listening).[4]

"There are four classes of sound protocols for misophonia and all of them contain a component whereby positive associations are formed with sound. The protocols differ in terms of the extent of control the patient has over the environment, the sounds used, and the length of exposure.... Notably, the protocol must be tailored to the individual. Frequently, more than one protocol is used concurrently."[114] (p. 115)

With that background, we can summarize results of the two studies of TRT used to treat misophonia that were reported in this systematic review.[108] One study reported results of patients treated in their clinic for misophonia and/or hyperacusis.[114] Treatment for misophonia was effective for 83% of 184 patients whether they had misophonia alone or misophonia concurrent with hyperacusis. The second study was a case study (one patient) who received treatment based on the principles of TRT.[115] The treatment included retraining counseling, desensitization, and habituation training. The patient reported benefit, which was corroborated by a reduction in the misophonia questionnaire score.

Dialectical Behavior Therapy

Dialectical behavior therapy (DBT) is a type of talk therapy (psychotherapy) that is based on CBT but modified to address very intense, negative emotions (my.clevelandclinic.org). Researchers evaluated DBT for treating misophonia in a patient (adolescent female) who had numerous misophonic symptoms that included "self-reported rage associated with sounds of chewing and sniffling."[116] The patient had received six months of CBT involving exposure to trigger sounds, which was intended to reduce her anger. Instead, the exposure therapy intensified her rage. The researchers reasoned that DBT "may be more appropriate for those experiencing intense rage responses, as it focuses on acceptance of one's anger rather than reducing it through exposure. DBT may be especially salient for individuals who do not respond to CBT and those for whom exposure only intensifies anger."

This patient underwent individual DBT sessions, once per week for seven weeks.[116] The treatment "concentrated heavily on learning to be mindful of her rage and tolerate this emotion through acquisition of acceptance-based DBT skills (i.e., mindfulness and distress tolerance skills). These acceptance-based skills provided opportunity for change strategies focused on alternative responses to anger by regulating her guilt and reducing engagement in behavioral urges (i.e., to avoid and become verbally and physically aggressive). Medication was managed by the program psychiatrist (paroxetine hydrochloride 25.0 mg) to simultaneously manage misophonic and anxiety symptoms." As a result of treatment, her "misophonic symptoms reduced from extreme to moderate."

In another case study, the (adolescent male) patient's "annoyance had recently reached a high level of anger and rage, accompanied by an extreme, uncontrollable 'fight or flight' response."[117] His treatment consisted of counseling derived from "DBT (acceptance, mindfulness, nonjudgmentalness, and opposite action" and from acceptance and commitment therapy (ACT) "(acceptance, mindfulness, defusion, and values)." After 10 50-minute weekly sessions, the patient "reported no significant difficulties and a continued decline in symptoms."

Pharmacotherapy

Finally, this systematic review reported on the use of medications to treat misophonia.[108] "The most widely reported medication class used to treat misophonia was selective serotonin reuptake inhibitors (SSRIs)." SSRIs "are a type of antidepressant that have been shown to increase levels of serotonin within the brain" (drugs.com). Serotonin is often referred to as the "feel-good hormone." Use of SSRIs in these studies resulted in "complete to partial remission of misophonia symptoms."[108]

It has also been reported that misophonia symptoms can improve with drugs that are used to treat coexisting (comorbid) behavioral disorders.[108] This occurred with a

4-year-old with autism who was treated with low-dose *risper-idone* (antipsychotic), a 14-year-old with attention-deficit hyperactivity disorder (ADHD) who was treated with a combination of *methylphenidate* (central nervous system stimulant) and CBT, and a patient with autonomic symptoms (rapid breathing and heart rate, sweating) who was treated with *propranolol* (beta-blocker).

Survey of Patients' Treatment Preferences for Misophonia

An online survey was conducted with 141 parents of children with misophonia and 252 adults with misophonia.[107] The purpose of the survey was to determine the experiences and preferences regarding any treatment received for misophonia. The authors identified a list of 42 potential treatments, which they sorted into categories: medications, dietary supplements, lifestyle modifications, relaxation strategies, psychological therapies, audiologic treatments, and neuromodulation.

"Overall, audiology treatments and lifestyle modifications were both the most popular and perceived to be the most appropriate treatments. Among audiologic interventions, active noise cancelling (addition of sound stimuli) and passive noise cancelling (sound protection such as ear plugs or headphones) were rated as most appropriate."[107] (p. 8) The most common lifestyle modifications were "home rearrangement and modified event planning." At least half of the participants had tried psychological therapies, relaxation, and/or supplements. The most-used psychological therapies were CBT, mindfulness/acceptance-based therapy, and supportive therapy. "Findings suggest strong desire by participants to engage in treatment, though almost half described dissatisfaction with the treatment options they have previously pursued." (p. 8)

Recent Studies

One study reported treatment with high-dose *steroid therapy* (oral prednisone) for a muscular injury.[118] The 35-year-old male who was treated also experienced severe misophonia. The treatment resulted in a marked reduction in misophonia symptoms, which "remained stable over several months." (p. 1) The authors noted, however, that other patients in their clinic who took steroids did not experience relief from their misophonia symptoms. They also noted the significant side effects of steroids.

A case study was reported for the use of *metacognitive interpersonal therapy* (MIT) in a young man who experienced misophonia along with obsessive-compulsive personality disorder (OCPD) and avoidant personality disorder.[119] MIT is used mainly to treat personality disorders through the use of numerous methods to modify patients' maladaptive perspectives on themselves and others. As a result of treatment, this patient had "a significant decrease in misophonia." The authors concluded, "MIT can be an effective therapy for the treatment of misophonia." (p. 8)

Another case study reported the use of acceptance and commitment therapy (ACT) to treat an adult female with misophonia.[120] ACT "has demonstrated efficacy in treating various psychiatric disorders via targeting psychological flexibility processes." [(p. 374)] This patient completed 12 sessions of ACT, and results "suggested the potential promise of ACT as a treatment for misophonia."

A research group acknowledged the benefit of CBT for treating misophonia but noted that it might not address common co-occurring psychiatric disorders.[121] They evaluated a version of CBT that can target multiple disorders—the *Unified Protocol for Transdiagnostic Treatment of Emotional Disorders* (UP). The UP has been successful treating emotional disorders (anxiety, depression, trauma-related disorders, and obsessive-compulsive and borderline personality disorders) that commonly coexist with misophonia. This study was conducted in two phases. First, the 16-week UP protocol was delivered to eight patients, which resulted in a revised version of the UP. Second, the revised version was delivered to 10 patients. Both versions were reported to be acceptable by the patients who learned skills for how to manage their misophonia symptoms. The authors concluded, "These findings provide preliminary evidence that this transdiagnostic treatment for emotional disorders can improve symptoms of misophonia in adults." [(p. 1)]

Summary

The authors of the systematic review that is summarized in this chapter concluded, "there exists no single front-line treatment for misophonia to date. This systematic review of misophonia treatments highlights the significant lack of strong empirical support for any interventions for misophonia."[108] (p. 8) Their conclusion is not surprising given the wide range of treatments used for misophonia, the lack of definitive data regarding treatment effectiveness, and the lack of agreement regarding which medical discipline(s) should manage the disorder. It is therefore not possible to make specific recommendations. General recommendations, however, are reasonable based on the treatment studies that have been reported thus far.

Keeping in mind that misophonia is an emotional disorder involving reactions to specific trigger sounds (and possibly sights), the objective of treatment is to eliminate or at least reduce those reactions. Another concern is the likelihood of coexisting psychological conditions that require treatment. Until we have definitive data regarding effective treatments for misophonia, treatment generally should involve some combination of counseling and sound therapy. The counseling can involve any of the methods described in this chapter, with CBT having the most research evidence. Within CBT, many different techniques can be used such as counterconditioning and exposure therapy. "Third wave" psychological treatments, including ACT, DBT, mindfulness therapy, MIT, and UP have all been shown to be beneficial on a preliminary basis. The method of TRT provides a specific protocol—both counseling and sound therapy—for treating misophonia and has been used and refined for over 20 years. A variety of medications have shown promise.

CHAPTER 15

Treating Noise Sensitivity

As explained in chapter 9, diagnosing a noise sensitivity disorder presents a challenge because it so easily can be confused with common annoyance by sound. Further, noise sensitivity must be distinguished from misophonia, which is a completely different sound hypersensitivity disorder—although both are characterized by emotional reactions to sound. Misophonia is primarily associated with *certain sounds* that trigger the reactions. The reactions may be intensified when observing the source of the trigger sounds or by other visual stimuli (such as seeing certain people or observing certain behaviors). Noise sensitivity reactions are *only* caused by sound, and the source of the sound is usually irrelevant—*sound in general* causes reactions in people with a noise sensitivity disorder. And to reach the threshold of being diagnosed as a "disorder," the problem should have at least a "minimal but significant interference with normal life activities" (chapter 4).

The goal of treatment for a noise sensitivity disorder is for the person to be comfortable in different environments that used to cause emotional reactions due to the perceived noise. What exactly needs to be treated for a noise sensitivity disorder? According to our working definition of noise sensitivity (chapter 9), perceived noise can cause annoyance, tension, fear, isolation tendency, and/or anger. These reactions, and any other associated emotional reactions, should be mitigated by treatment. Successful treatment may also reduce health effects that are caused by chronic emotional reactions.[55]

The scientific literature has very little to say about treating a noise sensitivity disorder. It is therefore not possible to recommend any particular form of treatment. We can, however, suggest treatment methods that would address the various features of noise sensitivity.

Noise Sensitivity Associated with Other Disorders

Noise sensitivity often coexists with other disorders, which may be the root cause of the symptoms. These coexisting (comorbid) disorders should be treated independently to facilitate the effectiveness of any treatment specific to noise sensitivity.

Appendix E contains a summary of many medical conditions that have been associated with sound hypersensitivity disorders. Loudness hyperacusis is usually suspected, but noise sensitivity is the more accurate diagnosis in some cases. Medical conditions that may be more likely to be associated with noise sensitivity include schizophrenia,[54] migraine,[122] traumatic brain injury (TBI),[123,124] multiple chemical sensitivity,[125] Williams syndrome,[126] autism spectrum disorders,[127] and post-traumatic stress disorder (PTSD).[58]

Identifying sound hypersensitivity disorders secondary to (or comorbid with) a medical condition is not normally practiced by clinicians (because of lack of awareness). With TBI, for example, there is the need to address all types of auditory deficits "that occur secondary to head injury, and yet, often go unnoticed by health care professionals."[128] (p. 2) This situation is due to a general lack of awareness about sound hypersensitivity disorders as well as inconsistent terminology to describe the disorders. Accurate diagnosis is of course critical to target treatment most appropriately.

Cognitive Behavioral Therapy

Reducing emotional reactions that occur when exposed to perceived noise is the primary focus of treatment for noise sensitivity. These emotions generally center around anxiety, so any treatment for anxiety or stress would be appropriate for treating noise sensitivity. CBT has abundant evidence in the literature for treating anxiety disorders. It is even claimed that CBT is "the gold-standard psychotherapy for anxiety-related presentations."[129] (p. 318)

CBT tops the list of psychotherapies that are used for treating misophonia, as well as for treating bothersome tinnitus.[91,108] There is no question CBT can be adapted to treat noise sensitivity.

The basic premise underlying CBT is that thoughts, emotions, and behaviors are all interconnected—changing one tends to change the others.[130] The *cognitive* aspect of CBT focuses on changing thoughts to be more constructive, which can then reduce anxiety and other negative emotions. The *behavioral* aspect of CBT addresses life activities to increase positive experiences, thereby reducing anxiety and other negative emotions.

CBT is not a fixed (one-size-fits-all) form of therapy but can involve numerous treatment strategies. To treat noise sensitivity, patients can be taught how to frame their negative thoughts about the disorder in a more positive way. A dozen *thought errors* (also referred to as *cognitive distortions*) about tinnitus have been identified (for example, *all-or-nothing thinking*) and reframed into more helpful thoughts.[28] Addressing these same thought errors about tinnitus can be oriented around noise sensitivity.

CBT focuses on stress reduction by teaching relaxation techniques. One technique is *deep breathing*, which involves breathing in a specific pattern. Another technique is *imagery*, whereby the person imagines a calming and peaceful place. Many people are familiar with *progressive muscle relaxation*. All of these exercises can help calm the body, facilitate relaxation, and ultimately reduce stress and anxiety associated with noise sensitivity.[91]

The research on CBT is voluminous with hundreds of articles published every year that cover every conceivable application of CBT to treat the various types of emotional disorders, pain, substance use, chronic fatigue syndrome, obsessive-compulsive disorder, insomnia, bipolar disorder, etc. We have barely scratched the surface of how CBT can be used and all the proven applications of CBT for addressing chronic disorders. Any CBT practitioner can learn about noise sensitivity, how it differs from other sound hypersensitivity disorders, and how to adapt CBT to reduce a person's symptoms of noise sensitivity.

Other Psychotherapies

It is beyond the scope of this book to go into detail regarding other psychotherapies that can be used to treat noise sensitivity. We'll just mention a few, especially those that have been used to treat misophonia (chapter 14).

Third wave approaches to CBT are becoming increasingly popular as treatment for many health conditions, including misophonia and tinnitus.[120,131] Why "third wave"? *First wave* CBT used different *behavioral* approaches designed to change what people *do* (their behavior) to improve their emotions (mood).[130] *Second wave* CBT added *cognitive* approaches designed to change what people *think* (cognition) to improve their mood. Third wave CBT uses the principle that changing thoughts and reducing negative emotions are not necessary to improve a person's psychological condition.[26] Rather, the focus is on becoming more accepting of the disorder that causes distress.[130]

Third wave CBT includes mindfulness-based approaches such as mindfulness-based stress reduction and acceptance and commitment therapy (ACT). These latest methods have been used to treat the emotional effects of tinnitus.[132-134] They can also be used to treat the emotional effects of noise sensitivity.

Exposure therapy is based on the CBT model of anxiety originating in aversive situations.[129] These aversive situations cause the person to feel threatened, even in safe situations. The person develops anxiety and avoids the aversive stimuli. The therapist guides the person gradually and systematically in exposure to the aversive stimuli. Effectiveness is seen as a steady decline in fear and anxiety over time. Numerous adaptations of this basic method have been developed and used clinically.

Tinnitus Retraining Therapy

Tinnitus Retraining Therapy (TRT) is used to treat misophonia (chapter 14). The TRT *neurophysiological model* is the basis for providing counseling for misophonia—as well as for tinnitus and loudness hyperacusis.[27,81] The model, as used for misophonia, can be adapted to provide counseling that explains the underlying neural activity that is associated with noise sensitivity.

Both misophonia and noise sensitivity are characterized by emotional reactions to sound. According to the TRT neurophysiological model, emotional reactions are manifested by activity in the limbic system, which then activates the stress response via the autonomic nervous system. This same pattern of activity would describe emotional reactions that are associated with noise sensitivity.

The other major component of TRT is sound therapy. The type of sound therapy recommended for treating misophonia would be appropriate for treating noise sensitivity; that is, *active listening to pleasant sounds*.[81,113] In addition, a person with noise sensitivity has likely been avoiding sound, which would tend to increase gain in the auditory pathways.[33] General sound enrichment would therefore be appropriate for desensitizing the auditory system (reducing its gain—see appendix F). This combination of passive and active listening may be an optimal approach for using sound therapy to treat noise sensitivity.

Summary

As mentioned early in this chapter, the scientific literature offers very little regarding treatment of noise sensitivity. It is therefore necessary to draw from the literature that addresses loudness hyperacusis and misophonia to suggest treatments that can be adapted to treat noise sensitivity.

If a person is diagnosed with noise sensitivity, the first question is whether the person has a comorbid medical condition that might somehow be associated. An underlying disorder that may cause or exacerbate noise sensitivity is generally the first priority for treatment.

The person needs to be educated about noise sensitivity, how it differs from other sound hypersensitivity disorders, and how it can be treated. The education should include the use of hearing protection (earplugs and/or earmuffs), when and how it should be used, and how to avoid overprotection that can increase gain in the auditory pathways and exacerbate the problem (chapter 12 and appendix F).

Various types of psychotherapy can be used, mainly to address the emotional reactions that define the disorder. CBT and third wave CBT are well-established methods, and other methods may also be effective. CBT for anxiety has been shown to be effective using an internet-delivery format.[135]

Sound therapy should also be part of treatment, with the same goal as for psychotherapy—to reduce the emotional reactions. It is generally a prudent approach that sound therapy should involve both active listening to sounds that are pleasurable (to associate sound with pleasant experiences) and passive listening 24/7 to promote a reduction of auditory gain to enable tolerance of increasingly greater levels of sound.

CHAPTER 16

Treating Phonophobia

Phonophobia, as defined in chapter 10, belongs in a completely different category than the other four sound hypersensitivity disorders (loudness hyperacusis, pain hyperacusis, misophonia, and noise sensitivity). Those four disorders are all characterized by *negative reactions* to sound, but in a uniquely different manner for each. Phonophobia is characterized by an *excessive fear* of sound—not *reactions* to sound. Phonophobia can coexist with any of the other disorders and is usually a consequence of the negative reactions associated with those disorders.

In chapter 10 we discussed *healthy* fear of sound, which would mean taking reasonable steps to avoid or protect oneself from sounds that are uncomfortable. Healthy fear of sound is to be encouraged. If the healthy fear turns excessive, then phonophobia is the diagnosis and treatment may be warranted.

Phonophobia is not normally treated under the assumption that it is an independent disorder. The underlying loudness hyperacusis, pain hyperacusis, misophonia, and/or noise sensitivity must be treated, which, if successful, may be sufficient to resolve the associated phonophobia. A decision therefore needs to be made whether to treat the underlying sound hypersensitivity disorder by itself or to also treat the phonophobia as a separate, but related, disorder. That decision would normally depend on the severity of the person's disorders (phonophobia plus one or more of the other four sound hypersensitivity disorders). If severe, then the combination of disorders may require separate treatment (in a coordinated fashion). If mild or moderate, then treating the phonophobia separately may not be necessary.

Cognitive Behavioral Therapy

If treating the phonophobia separately, then it is treated as a *specific phobia*, which is a type of anxiety disorder.[13] We have discussed treatment for anxiety associated with misophonia (chapter 14) and with noise sensitivity (chapter 15). We noted that CBT has been claimed to be "the gold-standard psychotherapy for anxiety-related presentations."[129] (p. 318) It is therefore reasonable and appropriate to use CBT for treatment of phonophobia.

Ideally, the person with phonophobia would meet with a practitioner who specializes in using CBT to treat specific phobia and who understands sound hypersensitivity disorders and how they differ. It is important to determine the person's relevant medical history to understand the likely source of the phobia and to target the treatment accordingly.

In general, relaxation/stress reduction techniques should be taught. Different CBT providers teach different techniques, mostly involving deep breathing, imagery, and/or progressive muscle relaxation.[91] Using any of these techniques to reduce anxiety is a helpful skill for anyone with phonophobia. Even if the practitioner does not treat specific phobias, any CBT practitioner can teach relaxation strategies. Audiologists who specialize in the management of tinnitus and sound hypersensitivity disorders also can teach these strategies.[103]

The *cognitive* aspect of CBT would focus on teaching the person how to think more positively and constructively about any sound that is feared.[94] First of all, the person should understand that these sounds are not harmful to the auditory system. They are not loud enough to cause damage to the inner ear, and they normally would not have any effect on the sound hypersensitivity disorder. That may not always be the case, however, as we will discuss next.

Can Sound Exacerbate a Sound Hypersensitivity Disorder?

It is relatively uncommon for sound to make a person's sound hypersensitivity disorder worse, but it does happen. Some people with *loudness hyperacusis* experience even greater sensitivity to the loudness of sound after being exposed to sound—their loudness hyperacusis is *reactive*. These people represent a special category with Tinnitus Retraining

Therapy (TRT), and the sound therapy protocol is modified to ensure that it does not have an adverse effect.[27,81]

With *pain hyperacusis*, exacerbation of the disorder by exposure to sound is a particular concern. With these people, any exposure to sound may result in prolonged pain.[37] It would therefore be inappropriate to tell these people that exposure to sound is harmless. These individuals represent a special category for which any form of sound therapy may not be an option.

Trigger sounds for people with *misophonia* are generally quiet sounds that cannot possibly cause physical damage to the auditory system. Exposure to trigger sounds typically causes anxiety and anger, and the emotional reactions may be intensified by repeated exposure. Treatment should reverse this effect to the point that emotional reactions are either minimal or nonexistent.

With *noise sensitivity*, exposure to normal levels of sound would typically be limited to causing anxiety but without any potential of causing physical harm. There are known health effects, however, in some people with noise sensitivity.[48] These health effects are caused by chronic stress and anxiety and not directly by the noise itself.

It should be clear how counseling differs depending on which sound hypersensitivity disorder underlies the phonophobia. An inaccurate diagnosis would lead to inappropriate counseling that could potentially result in exacerbating the symptoms. The greatest concern is incorrect counseling of people with pain hyperacusis because of the risk of causing prolonged pain when exposed to sound.

Exposure Therapy

This is a good point to discuss exposure therapy, which refers to gradual and systematic exposure to any sound that causes reactions. Exposure therapy is actually the treatment of choice for specific phobia.[13] This can be an appropriate method of therapy for phonophobia provided the exposure to sound does not exacerbate the symptoms, as explained in the previous section.

If exposure therapy is to be used, it is critical to fully inform the person as to the nature of the therapy and exactly what it will involve. The thought of being exposed to what is the source of the phobia can invoke anxiety; thus, any discussion about this approach needs to be compassionate and sensitive to the person's feelings about the matter. Patients should never be pressured to undergo exposure therapy. They should understand the rationale for why it can be effective, but whether they receive it is entirely their decision.

Exposure therapy can be done with the actual sounds that are offensive, or it can be done using recordings of those sounds. It would be preferable to start with the recordings and to play them at an extremely low level to start. Using recordings enables precise control over the level of the sound, which is critical when just starting out. Once the person has fully acclimated to the low-level recording, then it can be increased very slightly. Incremental increases would continue until the person can tolerate the recorded sounds at a reasonable level. At that point, the person can be exposed to the sounds in a live environment. Earplugs or earmuffs should be immediately available for use in case the sound causes significant discomfort.

Internet- and Mobile-Based Treatments

A systematic review of nine studies that used internet- or mobile-based programs was conducted to determine the effectiveness of this approach in treating anxiety associated with specific phobia.[13] Exposure therapy was the main component used by all of the treatments. Most of the treatments included therapist support, either by phone or email. Results showed that treatment was beneficial in most of the studies.

Although no internet- or mobile-based treatment currently exists for phonophobia, internet-based CBT has been developed and tested as treatment for tinnitus alone or tinnitus combined with hyperacusis and/or misophonia.[136] This preliminary study showed promising results for a similar approach to treat all sound hypersensitivity disorders, including phonophobia.

Summary

As for noise sensitivity, the research literature pertaining to treatment of phonophobia is sparse. We are therefore limited in describing some treatment options. Key principles can be derived from what is known about treating the other sound hypersensitivity disorders and about treating specific phobias.

As mentioned, phonophobia is in its own category relative to the four other sound hypersensitivity disorders. Those disorders involve adverse reactions to sound while phonophobia involves excessive fear of sound. It is essential to know what sound hypersensitivity disorder, or combination of disorders, the person experiences. Successful treatment of the underlying disorder(s) will result in the phonophobia becoming minimized or eradicated. It is essential to decide whether phonophobia should be treated as a separate disorder or to focus on treating the underlying sound hypersensitivity disorder(s). This is a clinical judgment that requires both patient and practitioners to be fully informed with an accurate diagnosis, complete history of the disorder (especially its onset), and thorough description of any symptoms experienced.

Because phonophobia is a phobia, the main symptom to be treated is anxiety. CBT is commonly used to treat anxiety associated with all kinds of conditions and therefore would be an appropriate choice for treatment. We've also discussed third wave CBT approaches, which may be appropriate. Third wave approaches, however, typically involve acceptance of the offending sounds, which is akin to exposure therapy. All of the caveats described for exposure therapy would therefore apply when using mindfulness-based treatment, acceptance and commitment therapy (ACT), and other similar therapies.

Exposure therapy should be used if at all possible to treat phonophobia. The goals of treatment are to mitigate the disorder itself and also to eliminate the unhealthy fear associated with the disorder. It's a balancing act to know exactly what to do, and no one method can be assumed to work for everyone.

PART 5

Wrap-Up

CHAPTER 17

Summary, Suggestions, and Resources

Summary

This book addresses assessment, diagnosis, and treatment of all five sound hypersensitivity disorders. This is a young field of study with an evolving understanding of the disorders and how they differ. The contents of the book are based primarily on the scientific literature pertaining to the disorders.

Much has been written about hyperacusis and misophonia. Unfortunately, "hyperacusis" is often used as an umbrella term covering all sound hypersensitivity disorders. Progress in this field will continue to be hindered until terminology and definitions relating to the different disorders achieve general agreement among the majority of researchers and clinicians who work in the field.

Distinguishing between *loudness hyperacusis* and *pain hyperacusis* is a fairly recent development.[3,5] The distinction has always existed for people who experience these different forms of hyperacusis, but many clinicians and researchers have only recently become aware of how and why they differ. The usual approach of sound therapy for loudness hyperacusis cannot be assumed to work for people with pain hyperacusis.

The term *misophonia* was introduced into the scientific literature in 2002.[42] Its Greek roots refer to hatred (*misos*) of sound (*phone*). Originally, misophonia was a blanket term for annoyance by sound in general.[9] Within a short period, the term evolved to refer to emotional reactions to certain sounds—mostly oral and nasal sounds. Interest grew quickly and we are fortunate to have an excellent *consensus definition* of misophonia that was developed by a large group of researchers in the field.[43] Misophonia is a well-established concept with ongoing research to understand it better and to develop and improve on existing treatments.

Noise sensitivity is a relatively unknown sound hypersensitivity disorder, in spite of close to 100 peer-reviewed publications with "noise sensitivity" in the title. It is defined by negative emotional reactions to sound in general, which is perceived by the listener as aversive "noise." The disorder is typically tied to environmental noise (traffic, aircraft and railroad noise, etc.) and its effects on human health.[48] It can be difficult to diagnose noise sensitivity because everyone experiences annoyance to some sounds. Also, noise sensitivity can be confused with misophonia because both involve negative emotional reactions to sound. Noise sensitivity has been erroneously referred to as "hyperacusis."[47]

Then there's *phonophobia*, which is in a category by itself. The other four sound hypersensitivity disorders are defined by physical or emotional *reactions* to sound. Phonophobia is a specific phobia—excessive *fear* of sound. It typically develops as a consequence of experiencing any of the other sound hypersensitivity disorders. Depending on its severity, phonophobia may need to be treated separately as a specific phobia. Otherwise, successful treatment of the underlying sound hypersensitivity disorder would normally be sufficient to resolve the phonophobia.

Suggestions

This book deals with each of the five sound hypersensitivity disorders separately, both for diagnosis and treatment. Working definitions are provided for each of the disorders, and principles of diagnosis are explained in chapters 6 through 10. The Sound Hypersensitivity Interview is described question-by-question in chapter 5. A good understanding of the different disorders and use of the Interview should be adequate to make accurate diagnoses.

With a diagnosis, the next step is to determine whether treatment is warranted and desired by the affected person. In chapter 4, different degrees of a sound hypersensitivity disorder (mild, moderate, severe, extreme) are defined. If the disorder is in the mild-to-moderate range, then treatment may not be needed or desired. If in the severe-to-extreme range, treatment is more likely to be needed and desired.

Treatment varies depending on the disorder, or combination of disorders, that is experienced. An accurate diagnosis is therefore essential. Pain hyperacusis is probably the most challenging of the disorders to treat, especially if the person experiences pain when exposed to *any* sound. The other disorders are more amenable to treatment, which generally consists of some combination of counseling and sound therapy.

Every person suffering from a sound hypersensitivity disorder should have the opportunity to receive effective treatment. How can that objective become a reality? It is first necessary that healthcare providers who would perform the needed clinical services (minimally, audiologists, ear-specialist physicians, and psychologists) receive training to learn what is currently known about managing these disorders. This could be accomplished if professional training programs in these disciplines were to provide the necessary instruction as part of, or to supplement, their curricula. Second, research needs to be conducted to establish an evidence base of vetted clinical procedures. Third, professional organizations that oversee these healthcare fields should coordinate efforts to ensure that clinicians are properly trained and qualified to provide these services.

This book serves as a call to action for all relevant parties to work together to achieve the goal of effective treatment that is accessible to all sufferers of loudness hyperacusis, pain hyperacusis, misophonia, noise sensitivity, and phonophobia.

Resources

Many clinicians are not likely to be aware of the distinctions between the different sound hypersensitivity disorders, nor how to conduct an assessment and provide targeted treatment. This book helps bridge that gap, and the references provided throughout comprise a fairly comprehensive body of information to learn more about each disorder.

There is no single resource to provide further information about all five of the sound hypersensitivity disorders. It is necessary to read the individual publications and the books that are available. Websites are not particularly helpful because of their inconsistency in terms and definitions and a general lack of understanding all the disorders and how they differ.

Many patients find helpful support from other patients in various patient support groups. Facebook, Reddit, and Discord are three popular social media platforms that offer multiple options for patient support groups with sound hypersensitivity disorders. For each social media platform, search on "misophonia," "hyperacusis," and other sound hypersensitivity terms to find and join current, active patient support groups. In addition, the American Tinnitus Association (ATA) website lists a number of patient support groups, many of which operate virtually with platforms such as Zoom and welcome patients from all locations. While the groups listed on the ATA website primarily focus on tinnitus, many include sound hypersensitivity as part of their mission.

Parting Words

Authoring this book was motivated by the need to make this information available to clinicians, researchers, and the general public. Since my retirement, I've written and self-published three books about tinnitus—the main focus of my research career.[26-28] Sound hypersensitivity disorders often co-occur with tinnitus, and I have learned about them continually throughout my career. Writing this book has enabled me to dig deeper into each of the five disorders by drawing from the relevant books and peer-reviewed publications.

It is my sincere desire that this book will contribute some clarity to a field that is young, unstructured, and greatly in need of evidence-based clinical guidelines. Research is picking up, albeit gradually, and there are bound to be breakthroughs with respect to both diagnosis and treatment of the different disorders.

May this book be of value to you, either in your practice or in your personal life. Please feel free to contact me via drhenry@earsgonewrong.org if I can answer any questions or provide any further information.

PART 6

Appendixes

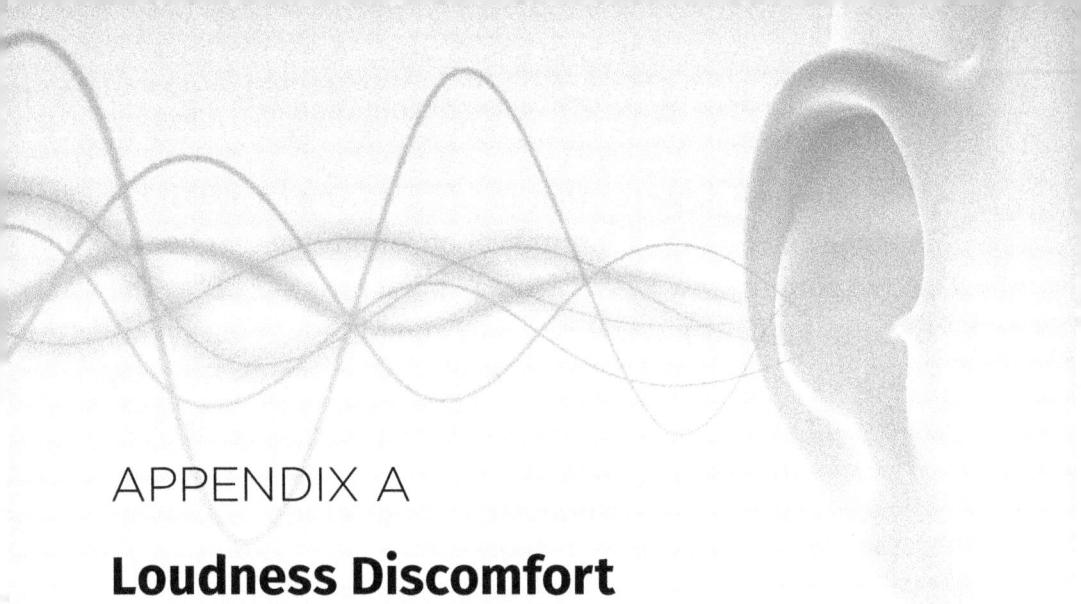

APPENDIX A

Loudness Discomfort Level (LDL) Testing

Audiologists perform loudness discomfort level (LDL) testing by slowly increasing the level of a tone or a band of noise while instructing the person to indicate when the stimulus is uncomfortably loud (or *about to become* uncomfortably loud). The testing is routinely done to adjust the maximum output of hearing aids to ensure that amplified sound does not reach the level that causes loudness discomfort.[137]

A person with suspected hyperacusis is often assessed for LDLs.[19] The testing can be done using pure tones at different frequencies (see Fig. C-1 in appendix C), or it can be done using a band (or bands) of noise. For example, the method of Tinnitus Retraining Therapy (TRT) measures LDLs at different frequencies.[81] With TRT, these measures are considered of "fundamental importance" in determining whether a person has a sound hypersensitivity disorder.

It has been reported that 100 dB Hearing Level (HL) is the approximate maximum level of sound that can be tolerated comfortably by the average person, as shown by the LDLs in appendix C (Fig. C-1A).[138] Loudness hyperacusis would be expected if LDLs are below about 100 dB HL. The lower the LDLs, the more likely it is the person has loudness hyperacusis. For example, Figure C-1B shows LDLs of 70 dB HL at all frequencies, which strongly suggests this person has loudness hyperacusis.

For a number of reasons, however, LDL testing is not normally recommended.[4] Perhaps most importantly, studies have shown that LDLs do not necessarily predict a sound hypersensitivity disorder.[20-22] These studies revealed that "LDLs cannot be relied upon to accurately represent a person's ability to tolerate sound in daily life."[4] (p. 519) This deficiency could be because of the variability in how the testing is conducted between different sites—standardized procedures for LDL testing do not exist.

Another concern with LDL testing is that any coexisting tinnitus (which is likely) might be made worse as a result of the testing.[4] Further, people with a complaint of sound hypersensitivity who are tested for LDLs are those who would be least likely to be comfortable with such testing.[19]

"It's an unreliable test that can vary among clinicians simply based on the instructions used to complete the task. I also find that most people in pain are scared to do the LDL test, and I don't blame them. I also worry that some individuals with delayed pain might end up being reinjured by an LDL test."[5]

Because of all these concerns, it is difficult to justify testing routinely for LDLs. The best gauge for determining the severity of any type of sound hypersensitivity disorder is to obtain responses from a structured interview.[4] The interview I recommend is the Sound Hypersensitivity Interview (described in chapter 5) that can be used to distinguish between all five of the sound hypersensitivity disorders.

APPENDIX B

Sound Hypersensitivity Questionnaires

This book would not be complete without listing and summarizing the different questionnaires that are available to evaluate sound hypersensitivity disorders. A main concern with all of these questionnaires is their inability to differentiate between the different disorders. If a disorder is identified, then one of the questionnaires might be appropriate to determine how much the person's life is impacted by that specific disorder.

Hyperacusis Questionnaires

Hyperacusis Questionnaire (HQ)

The most commonly used measure for assessing hyperacusis is the 14-question HQ.[139] The authors define hyperacusis as "a marked intolerance to ordinary environmental sounds." [(p. 436)] That is a definition of sound hypersensitivity in general, and hence the HQ was not specifically designed to assess loudness hyperacusis and pain hyperacusis. In fact, none of the questions asks about pain. The three dimensions assessed by the HQ are *attentional, social,* and *emotional.*

The HQ was originally tested with 201 individuals selected randomly from the general population, regardless of whether they had hyperacusis.[139] Another group evaluated the HQ with 264 participants in a tinnitus research study and concluded the HQ did "not accurately assess hypersensitivity to sound in a tinnitus population."[140]

A further study compared the HQ and the Noise Sensitivity Scale (NSS—described further below) in two diverse samples of about 100 subjects each.[47] Results suggested "a significant overlap between noise sensitivity and hyperacusis. The results underscore that NSS and HQ should not be used interchangeably, as they aim to measure distinct constructs, however to what extent they actually do remains to be determined." [(p. 1)] Finally, it should be noted that the HQ still has not been validated with hyperacusis patients.

Questionnaire on Hypersensitivity to Sound (QHS)

The QHS is a brief instrument (15 questions) that was developed and validated in German, using 226 patients who had both hypersensitivity to sound and chronic tinnitus.[141] The initial study determined that three dimensions were assessed by the QHS: *cognitive reactions, emotional reactions,* and *somatic behavior.*

The QHS (German version) was tested with 91 inpatients who had both tinnitus and hyperacusis.[142] They compared the QHS to three "other methods of assessing hyperacusis" and found "small to moderate correlations." Four of the items had "particularly low correlations." The QHS has not been tested in a population of people with diagnosed hyperacusis. Although an English translation is available, it has not been validated for clinical or research use.[140]

Multiple-Activity Scale for Hyperacusis (MASH)

The MASH was tested along with a hyperacusis-annoyance scale of 0 to 10 in a group of 249 "tinnitus patients."[143] The questionnaire mentions 14 places or activities, such as shopping centers and concerts, where discomfort caused by noise may be experienced. The strong correlation between MASH scores and the annoyance scale indicated that the MASH was sensitive to annoyance associated with hyperacusis in a tinnitus population.

Inventory of Hyperacusis Symptoms (IHS)

The IHS was first published in 2018 with the goal "to create a new scale that is reliable, valid, brief, and easy to score."[144] (p. 1025) The 25-item scale was completed online by 450 members of tinnitus and hyperacusis support groups. The authors reported that analyses revealed "sound statistical properties" and the IHS differentiates between subtypes of loudness, pain, annoyance, and fear. They also reported that a score of at least 69 (out of 100) suggested a diagnosis of hyperacusis.

A separate research group noted limitations of the original study to develop and validate the IHS: The participants (1) may not have been representative of patients treated for hyperacusis; (2) did not have their hearing tested; (3) did not have any other measures of the severity of hyperacusis; and (4) were not evaluated for tinnitus severity with a validated questionnaire.[145] This new study addressed these limitations to evaluate the IHS by looking at data from the "records of 100 consecutive patients who sought help for tinnitus and/or hyperacusis from an audiology clinic in the United Kingdom." [(p. 917)] They confirmed the statistical validity of the IHS but also noted that the scores obtained might partly reflect any co-occurring symptoms of tinnitus, anxiety, and depression—possibly reducing the validity of the IHS. They also proposed that a score of at least 56 (rather than 69) suggested a diagnosis of hyperacusis.

Hyperacusis Handicap Questionnaire (HHQ)

The HHQ was developed specifically to address sound hypersensitivity in the indigenous Indian population of patients with tinnitus.[146] Most of the questionnaire's 25 questions addressed "functional," "social," and "emotional" aspects of sound intolerance. The questionnaire was evaluated with 77 patients who had "hyperacusis associated with tinnitus." Analysis of the data suggested the "HHQ is a validated tool" for assessing hyperacusis.

Hyperacusis Impact Questionnaire (HIQ) and Sound Sensitivity Symptoms Questionnaire (SSSQ)

The authors pointed out that the severity of symptoms of any condition is different from the degree to which the condition impacts the person's life.[147] They used the example of two people with the same degree (severity) of hearing loss—one person's life is minimally impacted by the hearing loss while the other's is greatly impacted. In order to guide treatment efforts, therefore, it is important to measure separately the severity and the life impact of the symptoms.

The authors mentioned two validated hyperacusis questionnaires, the HQ and the IHS (described above).[147] Their concern with these questionnaires was that they measure both the severity and impact of hyperacusis, making it difficult to distinguish between the two constructs. A further concern was that some of the questions in the HQ are not specific to hyperacusis. The authors therefore developed two brief questionnaires, the SSSQ to assess the severity of hyperacusis, and the HIQ to assess the impact of hyperacusis.

The five questions in the SSSQ were designed to assess the type and severity of sound hypersensitivity complaints consistent with Tyler et al.'s categories of loudness hyperacusis, annoyance hyperacusis, fear hyperacusis, and pain hyperacusis.[2]

The HIQ contains five questions that focus on the degree of life impact due to hyperacusis. These questions were chosen to be consistent with some of the questions in the HQ and IHS. "There is no widely accepted gold standard for the assessment of the impact of hyperacusis. The HIQ was intended to remedy this gap by solely assessing the impact of hyperacusis, without dilution or contamination by other constructs such as hearing difficulty and severity of sound sensitivity symptoms."[147] (p. 255)

The HIQ and SSSQ were evaluated in a group of 226 patients from the authors' tinnitus and hyperacusis clinic in the United Kingdom.[147] All of the patients had tinnitus, and about 30% also had hyperacusis. Patients completed the questionnaires in the clinic waiting area. They also completed other questionnaires that assessed tinnitus, hyperacusis, anxiety, and depression. Both questionnaires were found to meet high standards of statistical validity and were recommended for use in clinical and research settings.

Hyperacusis Assessment Questionnaire (HAQ)

These authors noted that "the field of hyperacusis is young" and has numerous terms and definitions.[148] Citing a recent and well-researched definition of hyperacusis,[16] they considered that definition to be highly subjective and "overly general." They believed the predominant feature in hyperacusis is "the perceived loudness of external sounds." They noted that there are many types of sound hypersensitivity disorders and that the term *hyperacusis* should be specific to reduced tolerance to the loudness of sounds.

Based on this reasoning, the authors suggested the most useful approach thus far was to categorize hyperacusis with respect to loudness, annoyance, fear, or pain—as proposed previously by Tyler et al.[2] "We think that the perception of loudness is the predominant feature in hyperacusis and is accompanied by a reaction at the emotional level (fear) as well as a reaction at the physical level (pain). However, in our opinion, annoyance is not a feature of hyperacusis; this instead refers to misophonia."[148] (p. 2)

The authors noted the lack of a "satisfactory tool to objectively measure" the complaints of their patients with hyperacusis.[148] They conducted this study to create and validate a tool capturing hyperacusis in the categories of loudness, fear, and pain. Using a variety of measures, they evaluated a group of 106 patients who had both hyperacusis and tinnitus. The HAQ was validated in this population.

Misophonia Questionnaires

Amsterdam Misophonia Scale (AMS)

These authors noted that misophonia was a relatively unknown condition with "no option to officially classify the disorder."[46] They suggested classifying it "as a discrete psychiatric disorder" although the condition had never appeared previously in the psychiatric literature.

The AMS was developed as an adaptation of the Yale-Brown Obsessive Compulsive Scale.[149,150] At the time of its development, misophonia was considered to be strongly associated with OCD. It has since been shown in a group of 390 undergraduate students, of which about one-fourth experienced misophonia, that misophonia is directly related to OCD as well as anxiety and depression.[151] "Students are one of the most important groups experiencing misophonia." (p 261) Other studies reveal conflicting scientific evidence, suggesting a complex relationship between misophonia and OCD.[152]

A group of 42 Dutch patients "who reported misophonia" was used to develop the AMS and to measure the severity of misophonia symptoms.[46] Half of these patients were males, and the average age of symptom onset was 13 years. "We found in all patients a similar pattern of intense anger when hearing certain human sounds, impulsive reactions, avoidance of cue-related situations, worry of losing control, and the occurrence of obsessive compulsive personality traits."[46] (pp. 2-3) Although the AMS was not validated for its psychometric properties, this study resulted in a list of proposed diagnostic criteria for misophonia:

A. "The presence or anticipation of a specific sound, produced by a human being (e.g., eating sounds, breathing sounds), provokes an impulsive aversive physical reaction which starts with irritation that instantaneously becomes anger.
B. This anger initiates a profound loss of self-control with rare but potentially aggressive outbursts.
C. The person recognizes that the anger or disgust is excessive, unreasonable, or out of proportion to the circumstances of the provoking stressor.
D. The individual tends to avoid the misophonic situation, or if he/she does not avoid it, endures encounters with the misophonic sound situation with intense discomfort, anger, or disgust.
E. The individual's anger, disgust, or avoidance causes significant distress (i.e., it bothers the person that he or she has the anger or disgust) or significant interference in the person's day-to-day life. For example, the anger or disgust may make it difficult for the

person to perform important tasks at work, meet new friends, attend classes, or interact with others.

F. The person's anger, disgust, and avoidance are not better explained by another disorder, such as obsessive-compulsive disorder (e.g., disgust in someone with an obsession about contamination) or post-traumatic stress disorder (e.g., avoidance of stimuli associated with a trauma related to threatened death, serious injury or threat to the physical integrity of self or others)."[46] (p. 3)

Misophonia Questionnaire (MQ)

The MQ was developed by a group of experts who relied on their own clinical experience and a review of the literature.[153] It was tested in a group of 483 undergraduate students of psychology. The MQ contains two subscales—one identifies and quantifies the types of trigger sounds, and the other measures emotional and behavioral responses to those sounds. A final question measures associated distress. The questionnaire does not address physiological responses and focuses only on auditory triggers.[154] The MQ was criticized for being limited to a university sample and therefore not generalizable "to the broader population of misophonia sufferers" and for using only a single question to assess severity.[152]

Some psychometric values were validated, but because its external validity was verified using a questionnaire that assessed general hypersensitivity to sound, the MQ might not be specific to misophonia.[155] "The MQ was developed before the core details of misophonia were agreed upon, and therefore may benefit from refinement." [(p. 2)] Regardless, the MQ is widely used for measuring misophonia.

Misophonia Response Scale (MRS)

The impetus for this study was to develop and validate the MRS, which would address the omissions of "most current misophonia scales," including lack of validation, not addressing both physiological and emotional triggers, and focusing only on auditory triggers.[154] The MRS was not designed to diagnose misophonia but rather to determine the magnitude of both emotional and physiological responses to any type of trigger stimulus (auditory, visual, tactile, olfactory).

Three studies were conducted, using three separate groups of participants.[154] Study 1 identified an initial set of questions with the advice of an expert. The initial set of questions was reviewed and given feedback online by 247 people with self-diagnosed misophonia. The feedback led to changes for the second version, which contained 33 questions. Study 1 found the most common triggers to be sounds, followed closely by visual triggers. Smell was a common trigger, and a few people were triggered by touch. Parents were the most common trigger source, followed by romantic partner and colleagues.

For study 2, the aim was to develop the final version of the MRS using a new group of 366 participants with self-diagnosed misophonia.[154] After analyzing the data, the final version contained 22 questions, which included three subscales (emotional response, physiological response, and participation in life). An additional three questions assessed frequency, avoidance, and recovery time of misophonic reactions. Study 3 tested this final version with 482 people with self-diagnosed misophonia.

Statistical testing of the final version determined that it was "valid and reliable."[154] The MRS can be used with people whose misophonic reactions are triggered by auditory, visual, olfactory, and tactile sources. It measures both emotional and physiological responses to the triggers, as well as their impact on everyday life. The authors concluded that research is "needed to explore which aspects of misophonia have the greatest impact; for example, there is little to no published research that has established whether it is the frequency of exposure to triggers, the number of potential triggers, or the magnitude of responses that causes the greatest amount of distress and disruption for individuals with misophonia."[154] (p. 7)

Duke Misophonia Questionnaire (DMQ)

These authors argued that misophonia should not "be considered an obsessive-compulsive psychiatric disorder" but rather misophonia "may be likely to co-occur" with many different types of symptoms.[152] They noted weaknesses in existing misophonia questionnaires that included (1) relying on experts to generate questions rather than including sufferers and their family members; (2) limiting questions to those that assess "symptoms and functional impairment" and not including questions revealing responses to trigger sounds that could suggest specific treatment approaches;

and (3) inadequate statistical analyses. The DMQ was developed to address these limitations.

The DMQ was developed in two phases.[152] For phase 1, the initial questions were developed based on a review of the literature and feedback from expert professionals and sufferers and their loved ones. Phase 1 resulted in 377 questions that would be used in phase 2.

"Phase 2 involved rigorous psychometric refinement and validation."[152] (p. 4) Responses from a group of 424 participants were included in the analyses. This resulted in a total of 86 questions with eight subscales. The authors concluded, "The DMQ is the first psychometrically validated self-report measure of misophonia developed using a grassroots approach and multiple key stakeholders, iterative and rigorous analytic procedures to derive best fitting items ... and a range of features commonly observed in misophonia beyond severity of symptoms and impairment in functioning."[152] (p. 19)

Duke-Vanderbilt Misophonia Screening Questionnaire (DVMSQ)

These authors noted that numerous research groups had proposed criteria for diagnosing misophonia.[63] None of these criteria, however, was endorsed in the expert consensus definition of misophonia (described in chapter 8).[43] Further, the consensus statement did not suggest diagnostic criteria that would be derived from their definition.

The purpose of this study was to statistically validate the DVMSQ for diagnosing misophonia.[63] The consensus definition of misophonia[43] was incorporated into the diagnostic algorithm, which addressed the need to have a questionnaire that formally diagnoses misophonia using a standardized definition. "The DVMSQ provides a criterion-based algorithm to determine whether an individual reports all symptoms and sufficient functional impairment to warrant being classified as having clinically significant misophonia."[63] (p. 3) The diagnostic criteria of the DVMSQ are further consistent with the *Amsterdam UMC 2020 revised criteria for misophonia*.[156]

The 20-question DVMSQ was created concurrently with the 86-question Duke Misophonia Questionnaire (DMQ— see above).[152] Whereas the DMQ was designed to assess the many aspects of misophonia in detail, its purpose was not to diagnose misophonia. The DVMSQ is a relatively brief questionnaire specifically designed to diagnose misophonia and to quantify its impact on the person's life.[63]

The DVMSQ was completed online by 1,403 general population adults and 936 adults on the autism spectrum.[63] The total score was strongly correlated with the DMQ total score, and 7% of the general population adults and 36% of the autistic adults met the criteria for clinically significant misophonia. "This novel measure represents a potentially useful tool to screen for misophonia and quantify symptom severity and impairment in both autistic adults and the general population."[63] (p. 2)

MisoQuest

This research group pointed out the need for a new questionnaire to assess misophonia. "There is no fully validated questionnaire available that measures misophonia based on the current understanding of the disorder."[155] (p. 3) They developed the MisoQuest to meet this need. Its initial 60 questions were based on the diagnostic criteria that were specified together with the Amsterdam Misophonia Scale.[46] The MisoQuest was developed in phases involving 705 Polish participants (both with and without sound hypersensitivity) who were recruited via social media and completed the questionnaire online.[155] The final version consists of 14 questions with a total score of 0–70 (higher scores suggesting greater severity of misophonia).

The MisoQuest differs in many ways from previous measures of misophonia, including (1) it does not address symptoms associated with OCD; (2) it does not ask about the duration of misophonic reactions; (3) it is not limited to sounds produced by humans but to all kinds of sounds; and (4) diagnostic criteria include an immediate emotional reaction and the presence of anger.[155] Using this instrument, misophonia is defined as a condition for which a person is triggered immediately by certain sounds with anger as an essential, but not necessarily exclusive, emotion. The tool therefore is specific to the authors' definition of misophonia. The MisoQuest was developed in Polish, and the English version has yet to be validated.

Additional Misophonia Scales

Additional scales for the assessment of misophonia have been developed and may be available online.[152,155] They are generally unpublished, not yet validated, and/or are used less frequently than the other misophonia questionnaires. These include the Selective Sound Sensitivity Syndrome Scale, the Misophonia Coping Responses Survey, the Misophonia

Emotion Responses, Misophonia Physiological Responses Scale, Misophonia Trigger Severity Scale, Misophonia Assessment Questionnaire, the Misophonia Physiological Response Scale, and the Misophonia Activation Scale.

Noise Sensitivity Questionnaires

Weinstein's Noise Sensitivity Scale (NSS)

Purportedly, the first questionnaire to assess noise sensitivity was Weinstein's Noise Sensitivity Scale.[56] Prior to the NSS, questions about noise sensitivity were generally limited to transportation noise such as traffic, aircraft, and trains. The NSS extended the scope of noise sensitivity to include all sources of noise that might cause annoyance. The NSS contains 21 questions that ask about general attitudes about noise and how different sounds cause emotional reactions. The original German version was translated into English.[157]

It was recently reported that the NSS "has been used broadly in public health, occupational health, and environmental research, and has been found reliable in other contexts."[47] (p. 2) Further, experts in the field recognize the NSS "as the most used measure." The NSS does not diagnose noise sensitivity but rather has been used to categorize people as being either high-, medium-, or low-noise-sensitive.[60,158] "Higher scores on the NSS mean stronger noise sensitivity, but to what extent individuals with 'high scores' on this questionnaire represent pathological cases who would consult in the clinic, and what score is needed, for instance, is an open question."[47] (p. 8)

Noise Sensitivity Questionnaire (NSQ)

According to these authors, prior questionnaires for assessing noise sensitivity were limited to assessing overall (global) noise sensitivity.[57] To also assess how noise sensitivity affects different areas of daily life, they developed the 35-question NSQ. The five areas assessed were leisure, work, habitation, communication, and sleep. Two studies were conducted.

The first study with 66 participants showed that "the measurement of noise sensitivity can be restricted to a single measurement,"[57] (p. 23) and that a person's global NSQ score is independent of age and sex. The second study used 288 participants to evaluate the reliability of the global NSQ score, which was accomplished. The reliability of each of the subscales was good except for leisure, which might have been because the questions in that subscale "presumably did not cover the entire range of possible activities." (p. 23) The NSQ was also validated for distinguishing between low- and high-noise-sensitive groups for the habitation and work subscales.

Questionnaires for Assessing Phonophobia

Noise Avoidance Questionnaire (NAQ)

"The purpose of this study was to empirically analyze the relationship between sound avoidance and anxiety in tinnitus subjects with hyperacusis in comparison with tinnitus subjects without hyperacusis and healthy controls."[159] (p. 612) For this purpose, the 25-question NAQ was designed to assess avoidance of sound and anxiety in 56 individuals with tinnitus (with and without hyperacusis) and 30 individuals who had neither tinnitus nor hyperacusis. Hyperacusis was defined as "the experience of a normal acoustic stimulus as being extremely loud or uncomfortable." [(p. 611)]

Results showed significantly greater "noise-related avoidance in daily life" for the participants with hyperacusis.[159] The authors concluded the NAQ "provides a new instrument to assess the extent of avoidance in a patient and an outline of the specific situations and activities that are avoided by this person, which is useful for individual therapy schedules." [(p. 616)] Although the NAQ does not purport to assess phonophobia, the focus on avoiding sound makes it appropriate for this purpose.

DSM-5 Severity Measure for Specific Phobia (DSM-SP)

The DSM-SP[160] is not a measure of phonophobia, but it has been modified to specifically assess phonophobia.[63] The instrument contains 10 questions, which were not changed for the modified version. They did revise the instructions to say, "The following questions ask about thoughts, feelings, and behaviors that you may have had in a variety of situations. Over the PAST SEVEN DAYS, how often have you experienced the following regarding situations when you are exposed to loud or unpleasant sounds." [(p. 8)]

To make the DSM-SP appropriate for assessing phonophobia according to our working definition of phonophobia (chapter 10), the instructions need to be changed further from "situations when you *are exposed to* loud or unpleasant sounds" to "situations when you *fear* being exposed to loud or unpleasant sounds." That further modification has been made and can be seen in the Severity Measure for Phono-phobia in Figure B-1. It should be noted that this modified instrument has not been validated psychometrically. It can, however, be used to assist in determining whether a person has phonophobia.

(The Severity Measure for Phonophobia is available as a free download on the Resources page at: https://www.earsgonewrong.org/)

Figure B-1. Severity Measure for Phonophobia. Adapted from the DSM-5 Severity Measure for Specific Phobia.[160]

Severity Measure for Phonophobia

The following questions ask about thoughts, feelings, and behaviors you may have had in a variety of situations. Over the PAST 30 DAYS, how often have you experienced the following *regarding situations when you feared being exposed to loud or unpleasant sounds?*

During the past 30 days, I have:		Never	Occasionally	Half of the time	Most of the time	All of the time	Item score
1.	felt moments of sudden terror, fear, or fright in these situations	0	1	2	3	4	
2.	felt anxious, worried, or nervous about these situations	0	1	2	3	4	
3.	had thoughts of being injured, overcome with fear, or other bad things happening in these situations	0	1	2	3	4	

During the past 30 days, I have:		Never	Occasionally	Half of the time	Most of the time	All of the time	Item score
4.	felt a racing heart, sweaty, trouble breathing, faint, or shaky in these situations	0	1	2	3	4	
5.	felt tense muscles, felt on edge or restless, or had trouble relaxing in these situations	0	1	2	3	4	
6.	avoided, or did not approach or enter, these situations	0	1	2	3	4	
7.	moved away from these situations or left them early	0	1	2	3	4	
8.	spent a lot of time preparing for, or procrastinating about (i.e., putting off), these situations	0	1	2	3	4	
9.	distracted myself to avoid thinking about these situations	0	1	2	3	4	
10.	needed help to cope with these situations (e.g., alcohol or medications, superstitious objects, other people)	0	1	2	3	4	
						Total Score	

Summary

Clearly, no standards exist for how to assess and diagnose a sound hypersensitivity disorder. In this appendix, most of the different questionnaires that are currently available are summarized, and some are appropriate for clinical application. It is recommended to use the Sound Hypersensitivity

Interview for differential diagnostic purposes (chapter 5). The Interview contains items that focus on how a sound hypersensitivity disorder might affect a person's daily life by impacting everyday activities. With a solid knowledge of the different sound hypersensitivity disorders and how they differ, administering the Sound Hypersensitivity Interview should enable an informed and reasonably accurate diagnosis of sound hypersensitivity disorders. Any of the questionnaires summarized in this appendix would be helpful to confirm a diagnosis.

APPENDIX C

Loudness Recruitment

As mentioned in chapter 3, *loudness recruitment* is not a sound hypersensitivity disorder.[9] To explain, this appendix describes the concept of *dynamic range*, which is the number of decibels between the threshold of hearing and the level at which sound becomes uncomfortably loud. The dynamic range is specific to each frequency tested.

Figure C-1 shows an *audiogram* that would result from a standard hearing test. A person with "perfect hearing" can hear sounds at 0 decibels (dB) Hearing Level (HL). With hearing loss, the numbers get higher—the higher the number, the greater the hearing loss. The audiogram shows different frequencies that are tested (like different piano keys), from the lowest frequency (0.25 kilohertz/kHz) to the highest frequency (8 kHz). This audiogram is typical of a person with good low-frequency hearing and hearing loss in the high frequencies. Also shown on the audiogram are loudness discomfort levels (LDLs) at the same frequencies as the hearing thresholds. The LDL is the threshold level at which sound becomes uncomfortably loud (see appendix A). The number of decibels between the threshold of hearing and the LDL at a frequency is the dynamic range for that frequency.

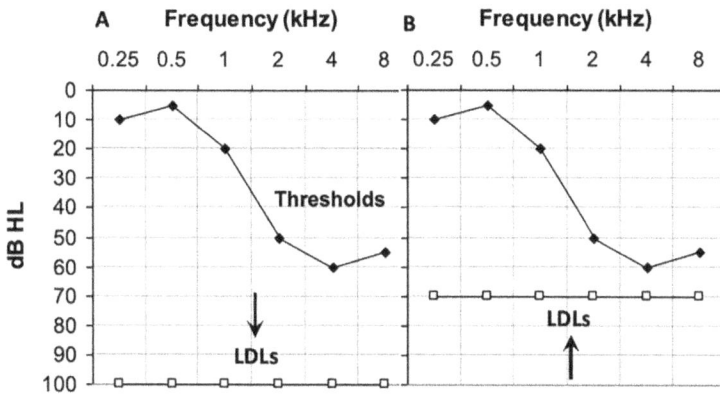

Figure C-1. Two audiograms side by side. The only difference is the loudness discomfort levels (LDLs). Otherwise, the hearing thresholds are the same—normal low-frequency hearing (5–20 decibels/dB Hearing Level/HL at 0.25–1 kilo-hertz/kHz) and impaired high-frequency hearing (50–60 dB HL at 2–8 kHz). **A:** LDLs are 100 dB HL at all frequencies, which reflects normal loudness tolerance. **B:** LDLs are 70 dB HL at all frequencies, which indicates reduced loudness tolerance and probably a loudness hyperacusis disorder. Please see text for further details.

The panel on the left (Fig. C-1A) shows a person with high-frequency hearing loss and normal LDLs. The dynamic range is almost 100 dB in the lowest frequencies. In the high frequencies, however, the dynamic range is *compressed*. For example, the dynamic range at 4 kHz is only 40 dB (100 minus 60). This compressed dynamic range is what defines loudness recruitment. The LDLs are all 100 dB HL, which means the person has normal loudness tolerance.

Figure C-1B is identical to Figure C-1A except the LDLs are reduced to 70 dB HL at all frequencies. Because of the reduced LDLs, the dynamic range is further compressed, which means loudness grows even faster than if the LDLs were normal. The fact that the LDLs are reduced to 70 dB HL is what indicates this person has loudness hyperacusis.

APPENDIX D

Development of the Consensus Definition of Misophonia

The term *misophonia* was coined in 2002.[42] A "consensus definition of misophonia" was completed and published in 2022.[43] The 15-member Misophonia Consensus Committee used a *modified Delphi method*[23] to achieve the consensus definition.[43]

The original Delphi method works on the assumption that a specialized committee will make more valid judgments regarding a particular topic than would an individual.[23] The committee is made up of people who have varying levels of expertise about the topic. The process involves repeatedly voting on statements pertaining to a definition until 80% of the committee agrees on the language.

The Misophonia Consensus Committee was assembled to develop the consensus definition of misophonia.[43] Following a systematic review of the relevant scientific literature, four rounds of voting were required to achieve the 80% threshold. (The third round of voting included a meeting of the experts, which is why this is referred to as a *modified* Delphi method.)

It should be noted that the committee agreed to refer to misophonia as a *disorder*.[43] "'Disorder' was ultimately determined to be a more accurate and useful descriptor than 'condition' or 'syndrome' for the purposes of the definition.... 'disorder' correctly implies the negative experience of individuals experiencing misophonia, can be useful in driving scientific inquiry to develop treatment models, and reinforces the professional and societal context around properly diagnosing, treating, and reimbursing care for misophonia." [(p. 12)]

The Committee published a well-thought-out and comprehensive description of misophonia,[43] which is shown in chapter 8.

APPENDIX E

Medical Conditions That Can Be Associated with Sound Hypersensitivity Disorders

Many articles and book chapters have been written describing medical conditions that are associated with sound hypersensitivity disorders. A thorough compilation of these conditions is contained in a book chapter written by D. McFerran.[25] In that chapter, the evidence for a link between different medical conditions and sound hypersensitivity disorders is reviewed. The author provides a list of 16 disease classifications, of which 60 specific diseases or conditions are described that have been reported to be linked with sound hypersensitivity disorders. He noted, "In many cases the evidence for a link is poor, based on case reports or small uncontrolled case series. The best evidence for conditions associated with disorders of sound tolerance includes hearing loss, tinnitus, and neuroses, though even here the evidence is insufficient to show causality." [(p. 127)]

This appendix contains descriptions of some of the more relevant medical conditions that could be associated with sound hypersensitivity disorders. The main point is to be aware of these conditions and their *potential* to cause sound hypersensitivity. It's important to always keep in mind that "research is hampered by confusing and inconsistent terminology and a lack of both objective and subjective outcome measures for impaired sound tolerance."[25] (p. 127)

Tinnitus

Many studies have reported a strong association between sound hypersensitivity and tinnitus. These studies show wide variation in how the two conditions are related, largely because of the inconsistent terminology. Most of the studies refer to *hyperacusis* as being related to tinnitus. The prevalence of hyperacusis in the general adult population has been reported to be anywhere between 3.2% and 17.2%.[70]

One study defined hyperacusis as "reduced tolerance to general everyday sounds.... in which the sounds are uncomfortably loud or painful."[161] (p. 2) According to that study, nearly 9% of the population experience hyperacusis, 90% of people with hyperacusis also have tinnitus, and the relationship is strongest when both hyperacusis and tinnitus are perceived as severe.

It has been reported that about 40% of people with tinnitus also have hyperacusis.[81] These prevalence estimates, however, depend on numerous variables. People will report the experience of hyperacusis according to which questions are asked, how the questions are worded, and how they interpret the questions. The reported percentages of people with tinnitus having hyperacusis have ranged from 7.3%[162] to 79%.[143]

Acoustic Shock

Acoustic shock (or trauma) was first reported by call-center workers who reported sudden, unexpected, intense sound through their earphones.[69,70] In response to the sound, they experienced symptoms including ear pain (*otalgia*), hyperacusis, phonophobia, imbalance, aural fullness, anxiety, hypervigilance, and insomnia. Otalgia is the most consistent symptom, which could be caused by the perception of pain due to activation of nerve fibers connecting the cochlea to the brain stem (as described in appendix G).

Because of the numerous symptoms that can result from acoustic shock, they have been referred to as a "symptom cluster."[71] The "cluster of debilitating symptoms" includes "tinnitus, hyperacusis, ear fullness and tension, dizziness, and pain in and outside the ear." (p. 1) These authors hypothesize that the symptoms are generated by injury to the tensor tympani muscle—one of the two middle ear muscles (described in the Middle Ear section below). Such injury could initiate a chain of events leading to elevated central auditory gain (see appendix F) and persistent ear pain. A thorough description of how these symptoms might appear following acoustic shock is available in the open-access article referenced here.[71]

Superior Semicircular Canal Dehiscence

The inner ear is a bony structure that includes the cochlea for hearing and three semicircular canals to maintain balance. The semicircular canals are looped tubes—one for each of the three spatial dimensions. The fluid inside each tube shifts with any movement, which informs the brain about the movement.

The *superior* semicircular canal is the uppermost loop. *Dehiscence* means the bony barrier along the top of the superior canal is abnormally thinned. This can result in hypersensitivity to bone-conducted sounds, such as the person's own voice.[163] It has also been reported to cause hypersensitivity to external sounds.[25]

Middle Ear Muscle Disorders

Some context is necessary before describing the middle ear muscles, how they function, and how they can be involved in sound hypersensitivity disorders. We'll start with a brief description of the middle ear and how the acoustic reflex modifies the transmission of sound through the middle ear.

Middle Ear

The *middle ear* includes the eardrum and the space behind the eardrum. In that space are the middle ear bones (*ossicles*)—a chain of three tiny bones that connect the eardrum to the inner ear (more specifically, to the cochlea). The ossicles include the malleus, incus, and stapes ("hammer, anvil, and stirrup"). The *malleus* (hammer) is attached to the eardrum; the *stapes* (stirrup) connects to the cochlea (via the *oval window*); and the *incus* (anvil) ties the malleus and stapes together to form the ossicular chain.

The purpose of the middle ear is to transmit sound from the air into the fluid-filled cochlea. To understand the task involved, imagine swimming underwater while someone above the water is trying to talk to you. The sound bounces off the water (because of an *impedance mismatch*), and all you hear is a muffled voice. Similarly, there is an impedance mismatch between the air and the fluid in the cochlea. The ossicles largely overcome that impedance mismatch. Without the ossicles, less than 1% of the sound energy striking the eardrum would enter the cochlea.

Acoustic Reflex

Two extremely tiny muscles are attached to the ossicles. The *stapedius muscle* (smallest skeletal muscle in the body[71]) is attached to the stapedius (close to the cochlea). The *tensor tympani muscle* is attached to the malleus (close to the eardrum—the *tympanic membrane*). The other end of the tensor tympani muscle is inserted in the Eustachian tube, where it "shares a tendon with the *tensor veli palatini muscle* suggesting these two muscles could be part of the same functional unit."[71 (p. 3)]

The purpose of the middle ear muscles is to facilitate the *acoustic reflex*. The acoustic reflex contracts the middle ear muscles, which stiffens the ossicular chain and reduces sound transmission to the cochlea, presumably to protect the ear from loud sound.[105] The acoustic reflex is primarily a function of the stapedius muscle.[164] The true function of the tensor tympani muscle is a matter of debate.[105] For example, some researchers believe the tensor tympani muscle is part of the acoustic reflex[164,165] while others believe it is *not* part of the reflex.[25,111] Contraction of the tensor tympani muscle has also been termed a *startle reflex*.[166]

The acoustic reflex is complex with respect to the anatomy and physiology involved. Only a brief explanation is possible here. Sound transmission to the brain starts with sound waves striking the eardrum, which is connected to the ossicles. The ossicles amplify the vibrations to the cochlea (overcoming the impedance mismatch), which converts the mechanical sound waves to neural signals that are sent through the auditory nerve into the brain stem. There are feedback mechanisms from the brain stem back to the middle ear muscles, via different *cranial nerves*. For the stapedius muscle, the feedback comes through the *facial nerve* (7th cranial nerve). For the tensor tympani muscle, it comes through the *trigeminal nerve* (5th cranial nerve).

When sound reaches a certain intensity level it triggers the acoustic reflex. That level is the *reflex threshold,* which is routinely tested by audiologists (acoustic reflex testing). Acoustic reflex thresholds are usually measured between 70 and 100 decibels Hearing Level (dB HL).[167] The acoustic reflex reduces the sound transmission to the inner ear by approximately 15 dB. As discussed below, abnormalities of the middle ear muscles are "hypothesized to be involved in the development of ear-related symptoms such as tinnitus, hyperacusis, ear fullness, dizziness and/or otalgia."[105]

Stapedial Reflex Dysfunction

The stapedius muscle is one component of the acoustic reflex, which also involves the cochlea, auditory nerve, brain stem, facial nerve, and ossicular chain. Dysfunction of any of these components can disrupt the reflex and prevent its activation to protect the cochlea from louder sounds. This lack of natural protection can be especially challenging to a person with loudness hyperacusis.

Studies have been inconsistent in determining the relationship between the acoustic reflex and loudness hyperacusis. These studies have generally focused on medical conditions that involve stapedial reflex dysfunction, including Bell's (facial) palsy (weakness of muscles in one side of the face), Ramsay Hunt syndrome (shingles outbreak that affects the facial nerve), and myasthenia gravis (autoimmune disorder that causes muscle weakness).[25] One study confirmed "acoustic reflex abnormalities in some individuals having hyperacusis."[168] (p. 501)

Tensor Tympani Syndrome

The stapedius muscle and the tensor tympani muscle have different roles, as indicated by the different feedback paths (cranial nerves) from the brain stem.[105,164] There is evidence that contraction of the tensor tympani muscle does not contribute to the acoustic reflex.[25,111] It is clear, however, that the muscle contracts during speaking, swallowing, and chewing, and when exposed to non-auditory stimuli such as an air puff to the eye, stroking the face, and head movements.[105,164] It can even contract when *anticipating* loud sounds and when stressed.

It is straightforward that the stapedius muscle contracts in response to sound and to vocalization.[105,169] The tensor tympani muscle does not usually contract in response to sound, unless it is activated by a startle response. "Contrary to the stapedius muscle (innervated by the facial nerve), the tensor tympani muscle is influenced by higher level centers of the brain and by the autonomic nervous system and as such is affected by stress, anxiety, and panic. It is activated by sound as part of the startle response, but it can contract spontaneously as well."[111] (p. 245)

Tensor tympani syndrome is due to a lowering of the *reflex threshold,* which is the minimum level of auditory and non-auditory stimuli that causes contraction of the tensor tympani muscle. Non-auditory stimuli include "sensory-motor activities in the region of the head and neck, for example, voluntary or involuntary eye closure; airflow to an eye socket; and tactile stimulation of the external auditory canal, speaking, yawning, swallowing, or chewing."[71] (pp. 3-4) The tensor tympani muscle "may also be activated as part of the trigeminal nerve reflexes (corneal and blink reflexes, jaw opening and closing, and head retraction."[71] (p. 4) "Importantly, a prolonged emotional stress or anxiety due to the acoustic shock (or other causes) may contribute to lowering the threshold of sound-induced tensor tympani muscle contraction and maintain this threshold at a low level."[71] (p. 12)

Tensor tympani syndrome is often referred to as *tonic* tensor tympani syndrome, which would imply a fixed state of chronic contraction.[166,170,171] The condition is usually one of frequent *myoclonus* (spasming) of the muscle rather than chronic contraction. One research group concluded, "our results are not consistent with tonic contraction of the tensor tympani muscle. Instead, they argue in favor of a hyper-reactive tensor tympani muscle with reduced contraction threshold.... The term tonic tensor tympani syndrome should be abolished and replaced by a more neutral term, such as hyper-reactive middle ear muscle syndrome."[105] (p. 30)

Possible symptoms of tensor tympani syndrome are numerous and include "a sharp stabbing pain in the ear; a dull earache; tinnitus, often with a clicking, rhythmic, or buzzing quality; a sensation of aural pressure or blockage; tympanic flutter; pain/numbness/burning around the ear, along the cheek, and the side of the neck; mild vertigo and nausea; a sensation of 'muffled' or distorted hearing; and headache."[104] (p. 1) Another author listed the symptoms as "episodic ear fullness; otalgia (i.e., ear pain); tinnitus; diacusis consisting of murmurs, clicks, and distortion; tension headaches; and vertigo."[166] (p. 250) Yet another author listed the symptoms as "fullness in the ear, pulsation, perception of abnormal hearing, feeling of vibration, dyacusis (various abnormal acoustic sensations, e.g., murmurs, clicks, tickling sensation, or may involve perception of distortions), tension headache, vertigo, dizziness, disequilibrium, and pain."[111] (p. 245)

These symptoms can be triggered by anxiety brought on by a perceived threat to the ear.[104] The perceived threat can be due to sound being uncomfortable because of hyperacusis. The condition can become progressively more severe. "For people with severe hyperacusis, pain may be constant or present most of the time, further increasing following exposure to intolerable sounds. For others, pain may develop for a period of time after exposure to intolerable sounds."[104] (p. 1)

"Sounds perceived as unpleasant or dangerous are particularly strong activators, and consequently, tensor tympani syndrome is triggered by hyperacusis and misophonic reactions to sounds. The presence of tinnitus, by general increase in stress and anxiety, further enhances tensor tympani syndrome. Misophonia tends to facilitate the presence of tensor tympani syndrome, which may become a significant, or even a dominant problem, particularly when pain is one of its syndromes."[111] (p. 245)

Migraine and Ménière's Disease

Migraine

A classic migraine headache is described as severe throbbing pain that usually occurs in one side of the head.[172] One of the accompanying symptoms is hypersensitivity to sound.[122] The hypersensitivity can start in the pre-headache (*prodrome*) phase and continue through the post-headache (*postdrome*) phase—thus potentially lasting up to about eight days. These migraine episodes are experienced by almost 15% of the global population.

"An association of hyperacusis has been made with chronic migraine headaches."[173] (p. 536) Sound intolerance can be experienced during migraine attacks and may abate as the attack recedes.[24] It has also been reported that sound hypersensitivity is experienced between migraine episodes and that it worsens during the episodes.[174] The literature generally refers to the hypersensitivity as *phonophobia*, which would imply a fear response. Such a label, however, would be inaccurate for what has been described as feelings of "discomfort or pain."[25] Sound hypersensitivity associated with migraine could be loudness hyperacusis, pain hyperacusis, or noise sensitivity. Completing a full assessment should clarify which of these disorders, or combination of disorders, would be the appropriate diagnosis. Of course, phonophobia could also be present.

Ménière's Disease

Although there is controversy (as discussed below), Ménière's disease usually has been considered to be a disease of the inner ear.[175] It is also referred to as *endolymphatic hydrops* (*endolymph* is the inner compartment of fluid in the inner ear; *hydrops* refers to swelling of the fluid). The swelling (expansion) of endolymph can disrupt the neural signals sent into the brain stem from the inner ear, altering both auditory and balance functions.

The symptoms of Ménière's are vertigo (spinning sensation), ear pressure or fullness (the ear feels blocked, clogged, or stuffed), tinnitus (usually a whooshing or roaring sound—like the sound of a large seashell held against the ear, or an engine), and hearing loss.[172] These symptoms occur as *episodes* suddenly and without warning. Each episode lasts for about 20 minutes up to a full day.[176] The time between episodes can be minutes or as long as days.

The precise cause of Ménière's symptoms is not yet known.[172] "It appears that although sufferers of Ménière's disease will in all cases have at least one ear with hydrops, not every individual with endolymphatic hydrops experiences symptoms of Ménière's disease. This finding has led to the conclusion that there must be another factor at play that induces those with endolymphatic hydrops to develop Ménière's disease."[176] [(p. 2)]

A current theory is that Ménière's disease may be related to restricted blood supply (*ischemia*) or other vascular conditions (*dilation of blood vessels*) that affect the delivery of blood (*perfusion*) to the inner ear during episodes.[176] "One such condition is migraine headaches, which appear to have a partly vascular component to their manifestation and have been found in close association with Ménière's disease."[176] [(p. 3)] Between 51% and 60% of people with Ménière's experience migraine headaches,[177] and up to 45% experience migraine symptoms during an episode.[176] "In our practice, we have found that the vast majority of the patients with Ménière's disease also have histories that are consistent with the presence of migraine"[178] [(p. 2)] even in the absence of a history of headaches.

Ménière's disease was named after Prosper Ménière, who was the first to describe its characteristic symptoms in 1861.[179] An additional symptom he described was migraine headaches because they occurred so frequently in his patients along with the other symptoms. He theorized that all of these symptoms had a common cause within the inner ear. This theory was studied for about the next 10 years but not again until the 1960s.

It is clear that migraine can be associated with inner ear disorders, relating to the vestibular system and/or the cochlea.[176,177] People may have purely vestibular symptoms, such as vertigo, motion sensitivity, and imbalance. Or they may have purely cochlear symptoms, including tinnitus, loudness hyperacusis, and hearing loss (even sudden sensorineural hearing loss). Migraine with primarily vestibular symptoms is considered *vestibular migraine*. Migraine with primarily cochlear symptoms is considered *cochlear migraine*. Migraine with a combination of both vestibular and cochlear symptoms is referred to as *cochleovestibular* (or *vestibulocochlear*) *migraine*, which may be considered the equivalent of Ménière's disease. The term *otologic migraine* has been used as an all-encompassing term for all ear-related symptoms including cochlear and vestibular, as well as ear (aural) pressure and pain.

Studies have shown an association between Ménière's disease and hyperacusis.[25,97,180] Cochlear migraine and cochleovestibular migraine may both be associated with hyperacusis along with other auditory symptoms.[173] Hyperacusis is not a vestibular symptom, and it would seem that vestibular migraine would not be associated with hyperacusis. However, in a study of 131 patients who met the criteria for vestibular migraine, hyperacusis was present in 90% of the patients during episodes and in 2.3% of patients between episodes.[181]

How can people with vestibular migraine also experience hyperacusis? According to Hamid Djalilian, MD (personal communication), migraine is a hypersensitivity in the brain that causes peripheral symptoms based on which area of the brain is involved. While vestibular migraine symptoms are primarily vestibular, hyperacusis can be experienced as well due to the brain hypersensitivity. This would be similar to a classic migraine headache patient who experiences hyperacusis (called phonophobia by neurologists) during a headache episode. In vestibular migraine, the peripheral symptoms likely occur due to a change in blood flow at the vestibular level, but the brain hypersensitivity that amplifies sound and light, etc. is still a factor.

If Ménière's is indeed a manifestation of migraine, then people with Ménière's can be effectively treated with therapies that are helpful for migraine.[173,176] The cause of Ménière's, however, continues to be debated. "The symptoms of Ménière's disease are likely a manifestation of migraine rather than an independent inner ear condition."[177] (p. 317) "Although there is conflicting evidence regarding the cause and treatment of Ménière's disease, current evidence favors it as a disorder of the inner ear,"[175] (p. 320) which may be due to a central (brain-related) phenomenon.

Traumatic Brain Injury

Traumatic brain injury (TBI) is caused by a blow to the head and results in neurological damage in the brain. The cause of TBI most often is falls but may also be motor vehicle accidents, assaults, and the head being struck by, or striking, a solid object.[99] A TBI can be mild, moderate, or severe based on the Glasgow Coma Scale.[182] In the US alone, 2.5 million people visit an emergency department yearly due to a TBI.[183] Mild TBIs (concussions) account for 90% of all TBIs. A leading cause of injury among military Service Members is TBI caused by blast exposure.[99]

The neurological damage caused by impact- and blast-related TBI can affect any and all areas of the brain, thereby having the capacity to disrupt motor, cognitive, emotional, and sensory functions.[99] Every component of the auditory system can be impacted, including the middle ear, inner ear, and central auditory nervous system. Even a mild TBI can affect the auditory system, with one of the difficulties being sound hypersensitivity. The potential effects of TBI are so numerous that "a multidisciplinary team approach to assessment and treatment is warranted."[99] (p. 154)

If a person has loudness hyperacusis, it can be assumed that it is associated with an abnormal increase in sound-evoked neural activity in the central auditory pathways.[96] It cannot, however, be assumed that the mechanism is enhanced auditory gain if the person has a history of TBI. This was demonstrated in a study that evaluated sport-related concussions.[184] Those authors concluded, "the type of hyperacusis found here is directly related to central biochemical, mechanical, and inflammatory brain responses subsequent to concussion." (p. 6)

Williams Syndrome

Williams syndrome is a genetic condition caused by a missing portion of chromosome 7, which can cause cognitive impairment, endocrine abnormalities, cardiovascular disease, and characteristic (elfin) facial features.[25] The prevalence of hyperacusis in children with Williams syndrome has been reported to be as high as 95%.[126] The majority of these children also have absent stapedial reflexes; thus, their sound hypersensitivity might be due to abnormalities of the acoustic reflex.[25]

Lyme Disease

Lyme disease is an infectious disease caused by bacteria transmitted by ticks. There are stages of the disease, and facial nerve palsy (one side of the face affected by droopy cheek or eyelid, eyelid won't close, lopsided smile) during an early stage can cause stapedial reflex dysfunction (described earlier in this appendix) resulting in loudness hyperacusis.[25] Lyme-associated hyperacusis in the absence of facial nerve palsy has also been reported.

Multiple Sclerosis

With multiple sclerosis, the immune system attacks and damages the protective sheath (myelin) that surrounds nerve fibers in the central nervous system (brain and spinal cord). This damage disrupts neural communication between the brain and the rest of the body. There is no cure for multiple sclerosis, and the symptoms and time course of the disease vary greatly between people. Hearing disorders have often been reported in people with multiple sclerosis.[185] Hyperacusis and phonophobia have also been reported.

Autism Spectrum Disorders

Autism spectrum disorders are neurodevelopmental disorders that cause problems with social interaction, communication, and behavior. The term *spectrum* indicates that these disorders are related but vary widely with respect to symptoms and severity. Autism spectrum disorders used to be considered separate conditions, including Asperger's syndrome (on the milder end of the spectrum), pervasive developmental disorder—not otherwise specified (PDD-NOS; in the middle of the spectrum), and autistic disorder (more severe symptoms).

People with autism spectrum disorders are often hypersensitive to sensory input—what they see, hear, smell, feel, and/or taste.[127] They experience sound hypersensitivity more than twice as often as the general population.[98] Their sound hypersensitivity could involve loudness hyperacusis, misophonia, and/or noise sensitivity. Depending on their ability to articulate what they are experiencing, it may be particularly difficult to make a differential diagnosis.[25]

A major study was conducted to analyze all of the studies on autism spectrum disorder that had reported data from which the proportion of participants "with current and/or lifetime hyperacusis could be derived."[64] In this *meta-analysis*, hyperacusis referred to *"loudness hyperacusis,* wherein sounds of moderate intensity are perceived as excessively loud, and *pain hyperacusis,* wherein sounds evoke physical pain in the ear or head at levels far below those needed to cause pain in a typical listener (i.e., approximately 120 dB SPL)." [(p. 3)] Their analysis included 67 studies (with more than 13,000 participants) that revealed the current prevalence of hyperacusis was 41% and lifetime prevalence was 61%. The study concluded, "our meta-analysis suggests that hyperacusis is extremely common in individuals with ASD, with prevalence rates greater than those of most major mental health disorders that commonly co-occur with autism." [(p. 13)]

Some co-occurring conditions have been noted in people with autism spectrum disorders.[98] For example, 29% of autistic people with hyperacusis were reported to have superior semicircular canal dehiscence (described earlier in this appendix) based on imaging studies.[186] Another study reported that the stapedial reflex (described earlier in this appendix) is delayed in people with autism spectrum disorders.[187] These kinds of coexisting conditions may prove helpful in the future for identifying people with autism spectrum disorders.[98]

Post-Traumatic Stress Disorder

Post-traumatic stress disorder (PTSD) is a condition of chronically high stress or anxiety that is experienced due to the intrusive and persistent memory of a traumatic event. A common symptom is *hypervigilance* (or *hyperarousal*), which is a state of increased alertness to all stimuli in the environment.[58] One of those stimuli is of course sound, and noise sensitivity and loudness hyperacusis would be common sound hypersensitivity disorders in people with PTSD.

A study of 300 US military Veterans who attended a tinnitus clinic revealed that 34% of the patients had PTSD.[188] Those patients with PTSD were twice as likely as those without PTSD to have sound hypersensitivity complaints. Another study, which was population-based, showed a higher prevalence of hyperacusis for those with PTSD compared to those without PTSD.[189]

Schizophrenia

A study was conducted to evaluate noise sensitivity in schizophrenic patients.[54] The authors noted that schizophrenic patients might be more prone to be affected by "stressful noises." Groups of participants included: (1) 14 with schizophrenia and auditory hallucinations; (2) 14 with schizophrenia and no auditory hallucinations; and (3) 19 controls (neither schizophrenia nor auditory hallucinations).

"The results in general indicated that, compared to healthy individuals, schizophrenic individuals were more sensitive to noise; furthermore, the patients with auditory hallucinations were more sensitive to noise in comparison with patients with no auditory hallucinations.... the response of schizophrenia patients might differ from that of other individuals due to their different minds and brain structures and their vulnerability to stressors. Moreover, this finding can be related to the neurological investigations that have suggested the likelihood of the deficient suppression of intrusive noises in pathways of the auditory nerves in schizophrenic individuals."[54]

Summary

In this appendix, a number of medical conditions are discussed that are known to have been associated with sound hypersensitivity disorders. The list is far from complete, and many questions remain as to the nature of the association in each case. It is important to at least be aware of the conditions and their potential to be linked with one or more of the sound hypersensitivity disorders so that treatment can be appropriately tailored to address the whole person.

APPENDIX F

Central Auditory Gain

An increase in *central auditory gain* is thought to be a likely mechanism responsible for loudness hyperacusis.[35,68] "There is a consensus building that hyperacusis is underpinned by an aberrant increase in central auditory gain."[19] (p. 359) For reference, I have written about auditory gain in some detail in a previous book[26] (appendix A) and in a peer-reviewed publication.[4] It is also written about extensively in the scientific literature.[1,4,19,24,33-35,72,143] I will describe the concept briefly here.

Central auditory gain pertains to the brain and how it processes sound. The auditory system must be sensitive to sounds over an enormous range of intensity levels—very loud sounds are more than a million times more intense than very soft sounds.[190] Changes in central auditory gain enable us to detect and process such a huge range of sound intensities.

How does auditory gain work? To simplify things, we can think of gain control as *volume control*, such as on a TV. If the sound is too soft, we turn up the volume; if the sound is too loud, we turn it down. Our brain does this automatically to adjust to the level of sound entering our ears.[36] Most generally, softer sounds cause gain to increase (the volume is turned up); louder sounds cause gain to decrease (the volume is turned down).

A study published in 2003 showed perfectly how sound and auditory gain are related in real life.[33] The study used two groups of participants. One group (*added-sound* group) listened to broadband noise from ear-level sound generators for two weeks. The second group (*deprived-sound* group) wore earplugs for two weeks. What happened?

- The sound generators (added sound) caused the volume control (auditory gain) to be turned down. This group was able to comfortably tolerate louder sounds as a result of listening to the sound generators.
- The earplugs (deprived sound) caused the volume control (auditory gain) to be turned *up*. Because of wearing the earplugs, sounds seemed louder than before—this group could not comfortably tolerate the same level of sound as before wearing the earplugs.

These same types of results have been observed in other studies.[74,75,80] Taken together, these studies reveal that auditory gain can be manipulated in a person by adding or reducing sound in the person's environment.

Loudness hyperacusis can be thought of as due to a person's volume control (auditory gain) being set too high. The person's volume control is hypersensitive, which means sounds are over-amplified. Ultimately, sounds that are comfortable for most people are *too loud* for the person with loudness hyperacusis. The general solution is to attempt to turn down the volume/gain so that sounds are not amplified so much. This can often be accomplished by adding sound, like for the added-sound group that wore ear-level sound generators for two weeks.[33] Wearing earplugs, or avoiding sound in general, has the opposite effect by making the person more sensitive to the loudness of sound (and less able to tolerate sound).

APPENDIX G

What Causes Pain Hyperacusis?

"In the most severe cases, hyperacusis is described as debilitating 'ear pain.' The response to trauma.... may relate most directly to such noxious hearing—'noxacusis,' to coin a term."[39] (p. 14723)

The purpose of this appendix is to summarize some causes of pain hyperacusis, or *noxacusis*, that are currently theorized. This is not a comprehensive review of all types of potential ear pain. The references cited are a good source for further information about noxacusis.

How Do We Experience Pain?

We have sensory nerves (*receptors*) located throughout the body that detect all kinds of pain. These receptors are called *nociceptors*. They detect *noxious* stimuli (hence, the prefix *noci-* for nociceptor and *nociception*) and convey that information to different parts of the central nervous system, which results in the experience of pain. Nociception is "the neural process of encoding and processing noxious stimuli."[191] (p. 3761)

Different categories of nociceptors are distinguished by their diameter, speed of signal conduction, and extent of their insulation (*myelination*).[192] Larger-diameter fibers conduct signals faster than smaller-diameter fibers. Also, myelinated fibers conduct signals 10 times faster than unmyelinated fibers having the same diameter.

"The speed of transmission is directly correlated to the diameter of axons of sensory neurons and whether or not they are myelinated. Most nociceptors have small diameter unmyelinated axons (C-fibers).... Initial fast-onset pain is mediated by A-fiber nociceptors whose axons are myelinated."[191] (p. 3760) C-fibers produce "the less well-localized, burning 'second' pain."[192]

Are There Pain Nociceptors in the Ear?

We need a little context to answer this question. In the cochlea, sound vibrations are converted to neural impulses that are sent into the brain stem via the *auditory nerve*. Sound vibrations are detected by *hair cells*, which are distributed like a piano keyboard within the snail-shell-shaped cochlea.[27,193] There is one row of *inner hair cells* and three rows of *outer hair cells*. Each hair cell is connected to neurons that converge into the auditory nerve on their way to the brain stem.

Type II Cochlear Afferents

The neurons that deliver acoustic information from the hair cells to the brain stem are different types according to whether they connect with the inner or the outer hair cells. The inner hair cells are contacted by type I neurons, and the outer hair cells are contacted by type II neurons.

- *Type I neurons* have large diameters and are wrapped in an insulating sheath (*myelin*)—both of these features increase the conduction speed of the neural signals. About 95% of the neurons in the auditory nerve are these myelinated type I neurons. Type I neurons "encode the information content of sound."[39] (p. 14723)
- *Type II neurons* have small diameters and do not have a myelin sheath. About 5% of the fibers in the auditory nerve are unmyelinated type II fibers. "In contrast to the predominant type I afferents that contact inner hair cells.... type II afferents innervate outer hair cells, which are more sensitive to acoustic trauma."[39] (p. 14723) "Painful hyperacusis, noxacusis, may be carried to the central nervous system by type II cochlear afferents, sparse, unmyelinated neurons that share morphological and neurochemical traits with nociceptive C-fibers of the somatic nervous system."[7] (p. 1)

Afferent nerves transmit sensory information to the brain. *Efferent* nerves transmit signals in the opposite direction as feedback to modify and control the incoming signals. A number of investigators have theorized that *type II cochlear afferents* induce pain to serve as a warning of cochlear damage.[39,40] "Type II afferents may be the cochlea's nociceptors, prompting avoidance of further damage to the irreparable inner ear."[39] (p. 14723) "Type II cochlear afferents may be not only acoustic sensors, but additionally respond to tissue damage as potential inner ear nociceptors."[7] It is known that adenosine trisphosphate (ATP), which is the source of energy in living cells, is also "a pain-signaling molecule that is released by damaged tissue, including the outer hair cells."[37] (p. 16)

Prolonged and Referred Pain

One of the symptoms of pain hyperacusis is prolongation of the pain. "Of relevance to hyperacusis, prior noise-induced hearing loss leads to the generation of prolonged and repetitive activity in type II neurons and surrounding tissues. This aberrant signaling may be the basis for the sensitivity of everyday sounds seen in hyperacusis."[194]

It is theorized that the extended ear pain that is often experienced with pain hyperacusis is due to inflammation. "As for somatic C-fibers, type II afferents could become 'sensitized' by prior trauma.... Undoubtedly the pathogenesis of hyperacusis must involve still other processes, especially considering that acoustically-evoked ear pain can continue for hours to days after sound exposure far beyond the minutes-long phenomena described to date. Such a prolonged time course suggests inflammation."[7] (p. 4)

In a study of 32 adults with pain hyperacusis, many reported *referred pain* in addition to their ear pain.[37] The referred pain was in the face, head (front, back, and side), throat, neck, and areas outside the head and neck. Many also reported that the pain could change locations.

Pain Associated with the Middle Ear

Appendix E contains a description of the middle ear, which includes the eardrum and the space behind the eardrum. In that space are the ossicles—a chain of three tiny bones that transmit sound from the eardrum to the cochlea. Two muscles connect to the ossicles, and when they contract they reduce the amount of sound energy entering the cochlea. One of those muscles is the tensor tympani, which connects to the ossicle that's closest to the eardrum.

The pressure inside the middle ear needs to be precisely controlled.[71] Pressure differences are sensed by mechanoreceptors embedded in the eardrum when the eardrum is stretched—causing a feeling of ear fullness. This sensory information initiates a feedback loop that causes the Eustachian tube to open, which ventilates the middle ear and restores normal (atmospheric) pressure. Blocking or dysfunction of the Eustachian tube results in negative pressure in the middle ear and the feeling of ear fullness.

The other end of the tensor tympani muscle is inserted in the Eustachian tube, where it "shares a tendon with the *tensor veli palatini muscle* suggesting these two muscles could be part of the same functional unit."[71] [(p. 3)] "Based on the anatomical proximity of the tensor veli palatini muscle and the tensor tympani muscle, it has been proposed that these two muscles form a functional unit controlling the middle ear pressure to maintain it equal to atmospheric pressure. The tensor veli palatini muscle is well known for its role in opening the Eustachian tube (which communicates with nasal cavities), allowing for the tympanic cavity pressure to adjust to atmospheric pressure."[71] [(p. 4)]

Appendix E also contains a description of *tensor tympani syndrome* (TTS; also known as *tonic* tensor tympani syndrome), which is caused by the tensor tympani muscle over-contracting.[166,170] This condition can result in numerous symptoms, including "sharp stabbing pain in the ear," a feeling of fullness in the ear, and other sensations that may be described as "painful."[104] "The feeling of ear fullness may result from the deformation of the tympanum detected by the mechano receptors inside the tympanic membrane due to TTM contraction and the dysfunction of the TTM-tensor veli palatini muscle functional unit."[104 (p. 4)] "Injury of the TTM can be associated with many other adverse consequences."[71 (p. 4)]

There can be numerous causes of tensor tympani syndrome. Prolonged muscle contraction (muscle overload) can lead to a cascade of events, eventually resulting in an inflammatory response in the middle ear, which "may lead to earache and otalgia (tingling and stabbing pain) as the middle ear mucosa is richly innervated with nociceptors.... The inflammatory molecules present in the middle ear cavity.... may further reach the organ of Corti and activate the unmyelinated type II afferent neurons synapsing with OHCs. These fibers are thought to be nociceptors signaling cochlear damage, by opposition of the type I fibers that transmit acoustic information."[71 (p. 6)]

Trigeminal Nerve

We have 12 pairs of nerves that connect the brain to different parts of the head, face, neck, and upper body. These are called *cranial nerves,* which help us to see, hear, smell, taste, communicate, and make facial expressions. The fifth cranial nerve is the *trigeminal nerve*, which connects to areas of the head, face, jaw, and eyes—to control movement of these areas and to sense pain, touch, and temperature. (clevelandclinic.org)

It has been noted that, while type II cochlear afferents may signal that tissue damage has occurred in the cochlea, this mechanism is only theoretical.[37] Further, "it is unclear how this mechanism alone would account for the referred pain and non-pain sensations (e.g., aural fullness, pressure, fluttering, muscle spasms)"[37 (p. 17)] reported by many of 32 adults with pain hyperacusis who described their sound-induced pain. An alternative hypothesis is "that overload or damage to the tensor tympani muscle in the middle ear can lead to pain that spreads via inflammatory processes to activate the trigeminal nerve and generate symptoms consistent with neuropathic pain and other otologic symptoms."[37 (p. 17)] Sensory information from the middle ear is transmitted to the brain stem. The brain stem center (*trigeminocervical complex*) that receives this information also has connections with regions of the middle ear, head, and neck. These connections could explain the referred pain that is often reported by people with pain hyperacusis. In addition, loud noise can trigger pain in people who have *trigeminal neuralgia* (disorder that causes intense attacks of pain in the face), which suggests connections between the auditory and trigeminal pathways. Further, these symptoms are consistent with tensor tympani syndrome (described earlier in this appendix), wherein myoclonus of the tensor tympani muscle can irritate the trigeminal nerve, stiffen the eardrum, or disrupt middle ear ventilation—all of which can trigger ear pain.

One of the branches of the trigeminal nerve connects with the temporomandibular joint (TMJ) and the muscles of mastication (chewing muscles).[71] This same branch also connects with the tensor tympani muscle (appendix E). Because of these connections, disorders of the TMJ may impact the tensor tympani muscle.

Summary

"Existing theories of the neural underpinnings of pain hyperacusis implicate structures ranging from the middle ear to the inner ear to the central auditory pathway. Middle ear models of sound-induced pain broadly suggest that over-load, damage, or myoclonus of the tensor tympani muscle can irritate the trigeminal nerve and cause pain in or near the ear. Others have shown that type II cochlear afferents share similar morphological and neurochemical proper-ties with nociceptive somatic C fibers and may transmit damage-evoked pain signals from the inner ear to the cen-tral nervous system (CNS)."[37] (p. 2) These authors concluded, "Taken together with existing theories and other surveys of pain hyperacusis, we feel that our results are most consis-tent with trigeminal nerve involvement." (p. 18)

APPENDIX H

What Causes Noise Sensitivity?

We discussed in chapter 6 how loudness hyperacusis is theorized to result from an increase in central auditory gain (see also appendix F for more details about central auditory gain). "The current understanding is that hyperacusis results from the malfunction of the central auditory pathways.... whereas the mechanisms underlying noise sensitivity are less well-understood."[60] This section provides an overview of some of the theories about *possible causes* of noise sensitivity.

Personality Traits

Noise sensitivity often results in *noise annoyance*. "Annoyance expresses mild anger, partly as a result of noise interference into everyday activities, coupled with feelings of invasion of privacy and lack of control.... people's annoyance responses tend to be stable over time suggesting a personality-based consistency to responding."[48] (p. 2) In other words, people with noise sensitivity are consistent in how they respond to noise, suggesting that their basic personality traits might help explain why they are noise sensitive.

Personality traits refer to a person's behavior, which is largely a product of the person's thoughts and feelings. The "Big Five" personality traits include *extraversion* (social, assertive, talkative—in contrast with *introversion*: quiet, withdrawn, avoids conflict); *neuroticism* (negative emotions are common); *agreeableness* (encourages positive relationships); *openness* (creative, imaginative, thoughtful); and *conscientiousness* (organized, responsible, efficient, productive, dependable).[195] These traits have been evaluated in people with tinnitus with the consistent finding that introversion and neuroticism (anxiety and depression) are common among tinnitus clinic patients.[26,196-198]

Noise sensitivity is thought to relate to personality traits.[47] Based on the Big Five personality traits, one study found that noise sensitivity was positively correlated with neuroticism, introversion, and extraversion, while another found it to be related to neuroticism and conscientiousness.[53,54] Regarding introversion, "introverted people show a low threshold for feeling noise."[54] (p. 77)

Regarding neuroticism (mood swings), "it may be possible that the central nervous system of individuals with neuroticism is normally under a bigger extent of arousal, so the crucial level of arousal in them could be more easily reached by noise than in people without neurotic tendency."[54] (p. 77) Further, "neurotic persons might show enhanced 'arousability,' that is, their arousal level increases more in stress. Additional unfavorable factors.... are worrying and anxiety, which might prevent them coping successfully with noise or some other stressors during mental performance."[54] (p. 77) Enhanced "arousability" is of course a common symptom with PTSD.[58,59]

Brain Mechanisms

"The neuronal mechanisms of sound processing may be the key to understanding the origin of noise sensitivity."[60] (p. 5) "Noise sensitivity is not merely an auditory phenomenon but instead has underlying neuronal mechanisms."[54] (p. 77)

"Noise sensitivity is associated with the structural organization of the brain."[54] (p. 77) One brain area of interest is the auditory cortex—where sound is consciously perceived. It has been shown that people who are continuously exposed to noisy environments, but without damage to the ears, may develop changes in how the cortex responds to sounds.[44,60]

It has been shown that noise-sensitive individuals have (a) reduced "sensory gating," meaning the auditory pathways allow too much noise-related neural activity to enter the cortex; and (b) enlarged volumes of the auditory cortex and other brain areas that are involved with auditory perception and emotional processing.[54] Further, it has been theorized that noise sensitivity "is physiologically related to the continuous arousal" of a number of areas of the brain.[53] (p. 179)

Genetics and Effects on Health

Some studies provide evidence that noise sensitivity has a genetic basis. "It has been shown that noise sensitivity has psychological and physiological components. It does aggregate in families and probably has a genetic component too."[54] (p. 77)

"There is evidence of an underlying genetic basis to noise sensitivity which could be linked to susceptibility to ill-health. Studies have repeatedly found largely cross-sectional associations with both psychological ill-health and personality traits such as neuroticism and trait anxiety. Noise sensitivity is also associated to sensitivity to other environmental stimuli."[48] (p. 2)

"Subjects with high noise sensitivity reportedly experience sympathetic nervous system activation in response to noise, release larger amounts of cortisol, and have chronically weak immune systems.... individuals with high noise sensitivity may be more likely to develop illnesses when exposed to environmental noise. This would support the stress model—a theoretical model of the effect of environmental noise on health—and, more specifically, the hypothesis that noise sensitivity primarily or secondarily mediates the occurrence of disease."[52] (p. 8)

"Generally, individuals who are older, female, and have a lower education or income level are more likely to experience health effects from environmental noise."[52] (p. 8)

"Significant differences in heart rate change or heart rate variability have been observed between noise-sensitive and noise-resistant groups, that is, sensitive individuals show more heart rate variability and other physiological reactions."[54] (p. 77)

APPENDIX I

What Causes Phonophobia?

Mechanisms underlying the development of any specific phobia would apply to phonophobia. We therefore turn to the phobia literature to address this question. "People who suffer from specific phobias work hard to avoid their phobia stimuli even though they know there is no threat or danger, but they feel powerless."[61] (p. 462) Why does this happen?

Conditioned Fear

One reason a person might develop a specific phobia is because of the experience of a traumatic event.[61] Any traumatic experience can result in a phobia toward whatever caused the trauma. The fear is associated with the event and is referred to as *conditioned fear*. If a person is attacked by a dog, the attack is the event that may condition the person to fear all dogs. The sight of any dog might trigger the phobic fear response that is associated with the event, which may have occurred many years previously. A specific phobia can last a lifetime.

Innate Fear

Phobias can also develop without being associated with any experience.[61] These kinds of phobias have been referred to as *non-experiential* and *non-associative* phobias. They are an extreme form of *innate fear*. An example of non-experiential/non-associative fear is a child's innate fear of darkness (*nyctophobia*). Fear of darkness usually resolves as the person grows up and learns that darkness per se does not normally indicate any threat of danger. In some cases, however, a child's fear of darkness can be sensitized such that the emotional reactions to darkness become exaggerated to the point of being a specific phobia.

Sensitization of Innate Fear

How does innate fear become sensitized? There are "fear circuits" in the brain, which are thought to be coordinated by the *amygdala*.[61,65] Normally, these fear circuits serve the purpose of detecting threats and thus serve as a protective mechanism. Dysfunctions in these fear circuits, such as a damaged amygdala, may occur, which could reduce the *excitability threshold* for fear—making it more likely to be fearful.[66] "For example, in most children, darkness may activate the amygdala. However, this amygdala activation may be exaggerated (sensitized) in children who develop nyctophobia, due to the pathological changes in the excitability threshold in fear circuits…. Sensitization-associated increased amygdala activity is a key amygdala mechanism contributing to fear sensitization in nonexperiential phobia."[61] (pp. 462, 465)

Lack of Habituation

In addition to sensitization of the fear circuits, there may be a lack of *habituation*.[61] Habituation refers generally to a decrease in responsiveness as a result of repeated stimulation by a stimulus that has no relevance to a person's conscious activity. Habituation must occur in order for innate fear to resolve. "For example, fear of the dark is often lost over time through repeated exposure to darkness without any harm. This may be characterized by a decrement of amygdala activation in response to repeated darkness exposure. A deficiency in this mechanism (i.e., amygdala habituation) may therefore contribute to the persistence of nonexperiential phobia."[61] (p. 462)

How Phonophobia May Develop

We can apply what's known about conditioned fear and innate fear to propose how phonophobia might develop—remembering our working definition: *Phonophobia is an excessive, persistent state of fear that either specific sounds or sound in general will cause discomfort, distress, or pain.*

Conditioned Fear and Phonophobia

Any acoustic event experienced as traumatic or shocking might result in phonophobia. Two obvious possibilities are *traumatic noise* and *acoustic shock*.

Traumatic noise is caused by sound that causes permanent damage to the inner ear—to the outer hair cells but possibly also to the inner hair cells.[67] Such sound would include exposure to things like a firecracker, airhorn blast, gunshot, or airbag deployment. These, and many other sources of traumatic noise, can result in immediate effects in the central auditory system, which can be manifested as hearing loss, tinnitus, and sound hypersensitivity.[68] The emotional impact of noise trauma clearly could result in phonophobia.

As explained in appendix E, *acoustic shock* can result from sudden, unexpected, intense sound.[69,70] The primary difference between noise trauma and acoustic shock is that the sound responsible for acoustic shock is "rarely sufficient to result in permanent cochlear damage."[71 (p. 1)] It can, however, result in "tinnitus, hyperacusis, ear fullness (feeling of abnormal pressure in the middle ear) and ear tension, dizziness, vertigo, and pain in and outside the ear." In some cases, these symptoms "can become chronic and seriously impact quality of life." Acoustic shock is a traumatic event with numerous potential consequences that could cause the onset of phonophobia.

Sound hypersensitivity disorders (loudness hyperacusis, pain hyperacusis, misophonia, noise sensitivity) may not be associated with noise trauma or acoustic shock. They may develop gradually and in fact may not be associated with any precipitating event. The repeated experience of any of these disorders, however, can lead to phonophobia.

Loudness hyperacusis and pain hyperacusis are disorders defined by physical discomfort. That discomfort, however, can result in emotional distress—ranging from mild to extreme (chapter 4). Misophonia and noise sensitivity are, by definition, emotional disorders, and the distress likewise can range from mild to extreme. It might be postulated that the greater the distress, the greater the likelihood the person will develop phonophobia. Phonophobia therefore could develop as a result of experiencing any of these sound hypersensitivity disorders due to the mechanism of conditioned fear.

Innate Fear and Phonophobia

Finally, some people might have phonophobia that is not associated with any traumatic event nor any sound hypersensitivity disorder. Just like our example of a child who fears the dark, a child or an adolescent might fear sound in general or certain sounds in particular.

We do know that sound hypersensitivity disorders can develop during childhood. Misophonia in particular is known to have its onset often during childhood or early adolescence.[45] Experiencing misophonia could lead to phonophobia, but this would be an example of conditioned fear.

Phobias in general might help to explain how phonophobia could result from innate fear. "Genetic, familial, environmental, or developmental factors play an important role in the development of this type of specific phobia."[61] (p. 462) It has been shown that noise sensitivity can be a genetic trait, with one study revealing an estimate of *heritability* (amount of variation in a population attributed to genetic differences) of 36% (40% when excluding hearing-impaired subjects).[199] These authors concluded, "noise sensitivity does aggregate in families and probably has a genetic component." [(p. 245)]

Noise sensitivity is commonly experienced by people with various psychological disorders, including anxiety, depression, and autism spectrum disorder.[11] Personality is also a factor.[47] These people generally have an innate "need for quiet," which can develop during childhood. Factors that predispose people to be noise sensitive are addressed in appendix H, What Causes Noise Sensitivity?

Studies of Treatments for Hyperacusis

Scoping Reviews

Results of two *scoping reviews* that evaluated treatments for hyperacusis are summarized below. A scoping review is similar to a *systematic review*. How are they similar? They are both done to determine what evidence exists in the scientific literature regarding a specific topic. They both involve a search of the literature to identify all qualified studies that are relevant to the topic and then summarizing (*synthesizing*) the results of those studies. How do they differ? Systematic reviews evaluate only controlled trials, while scoping reviews also include observational (uncontrolled) trials. Systematic reviews generally include a risk-of-bias assessment for each trial covered in the review, which is not done with scoping reviews.

Fackrell et al. (2017)

This scoping review revealed difficulties in determining what methods are effective for treating hyperacusis.[24] The researchers reviewed 43 published studies about hyperacusis. Only two-thirds of these provided a definition of "hyperacusis," and the definitions varied between studies. Different assessment tools were used to diagnose hyperacusis and to evaluate outcomes of treatment. Further, only five of the 43 studies were randomized and controlled, and only two were focused only on people with hyperacusis. The study provides abundant evidence of the need for standardizing definitions, assessment and diagnostic procedures, treatments, and outcome assessment.

The authors defined hyperacusis as "the perception of everyday environmental sound as being overwhelmingly loud or intense."[24] [(p. 1)] This definition would include loudness hyperacusis and pain hyperacusis. It could, however, also include noise sensitivity.

Of the 43 studies, only 19 "sought to evaluate interventions or management strategies specifically aimed at reducing hyperacusis. For the most part, the studies explored interventions that were primarily aimed at reducing effects of tinnitus. Management strategies explored were Cognitive Behavioral Therapy (CBT), Tinnitus Retraining Therapy (TRT), counseling, devices, pharmacological therapy, and surgery."[24] [(p. 16)]

TRT was the most commonly used treatment—16 studies, of which nine used "a classic TRT protocol" to treat hyperacusis.[24] For most of these TRT studies, "the treatment was beneficial to patients with hyperacusis." [(p. 20)] Three studies evaluated the use of CBT for hyperacusis. None of these studies used CBT alone—all of them included "graded sound exposure"; thus, it is not clear if benefit received (which was minimal) was due to the CBT.

One study evaluated "counseling alone."[24] Eleven studies evaluated the use of different devices that produced various forms of sound therapy for desensitization. Five case studies were reported for the use of pharmacological therapy. Finally, six studies reported results of surgery specifically for hyperacusis. Results of these studies varied, and more than half were "based on individual case studies and therefore cannot be generalized. In addition to this, management strategies were typically evaluated in patients reporting hyperacusis as a secondary complaint or as part of a symptom set, and as such the outcomes reported only provided an indication of effectiveness for hyperacusis. There is a lack of sufficient evidence to identify effective management strategies." [(p. 19)]

Kalsoom et al. (2024)

The authors of this 2024 scoping review stated, "Currently, there is no consensus on the treatment for hyperacusis. A number of interventions that have been reported in the literature include Cognitive Behavioral Therapy (CBT), counseling alone, Tinnitus Retraining Therapy (TRT)— which includes some directive counseling and sound therapy—surgery where appropriate, pharmacological therapy, and sound therapy using devices."[73] [(p. 2)]

The methods mentioned in this 2024 study are the same as those evaluated in the Fackrell et al. (2017) study.[24] The 2024 study, however, focused on sound therapy that is used for the treatment of hyperacusis.[73] The authors used the consensus definition of hyperacusis that was published in 2021: "reduced tolerance to sound(s) that are perceived as normal to the majority of the population or were perceived as normal to the person before their onset of hyperacusis."[16] (p. 607)

The review identified 31 studies that met inclusion criteria.[73] Participants in these studies described their hyperacusis as "environmental sounds, hypersensitivity to sound, reduced sound tolerance, and discomfort to sound. Several studies reported the emotional impact of hyperacusis, describing negative symptoms, reports of distress and social isolation, and the inability to use hearing aids." (p. 6)

Of the 31 studies, 23 reported using the TRT protocol.[73] The other studies used acoustic training, headphone/CD player, acoustic phase-out device, sound suppression devices, tabletop sound generators, and hearing aids/sound generators/combination devices. All of these methods, except for the phase-out device, resulted in positive outcomes. The authors, however, concluded, "There is limited evidence supporting the use of sound therapy for patients with hyperacusis. There is a further lack of evidence describing specific intervention parameters. Despite frequent use of the TRT protocol, further randomized controlled trials are required to determine the protocol's effectiveness in treating hyperacusis." (p. 10)

Tinnitus Retraining Therapy (TRT)

This study was conducted to evaluate the therapeutic effect of ear-level sound generators on tinnitus and hyperacusis, using the method of TRT.[200] Forty-two of the patients had hyperacusis as their primary complaint. In this retrospective chart review of clinical data, loudness discomfort levels were significantly increased for the hyperacusis patients after using the sound generators for six months. The authors concluded, "Sound generators with TRT seem to be an effective treatment modality for all tinnitus patients, especially those with comorbid hyperacusis." [(p. 135)]

Cognitive Behavioral Therapy (CBT)

An article summarized "key findings and conclusions from the Third International Conference on Hyperacusis," which was held in the United Kingdom in 2017.[201] The authors defined hyperacusis as "intolerance of certain everyday sounds that causes significant distress and impairment in social, occupational, recreational, and other day-to-day activities. The sounds may be perceived as uncomfortably loud, unpleasant, frightening, or painful." [(p. 162)] Note that this definition would include all types of sound hypersensitivity disorders. The authors did, in fact, state that the main topics discussed at the meeting included hyperacusis, misophonia, and noise sensitivity. The meeting focused mostly on assessment and underlying mechanisms of sound hypersensitivity disorders. Only CBT was discussed as treatment, with the conclusion, "Audiologist-delivered CBT gave promising results with regard to changes in hyperacusis handicap scores." [(p. 168)] This same basic conclusion was made in a study that analyzed data from patients who received CBT for tinnitus and/or hyperacusis: "Audiologist-delivered CBT led to significant improvements in self-report measures of tinnitus and hyperacusis handicap and insomnia."[101] (p. 547)

A review was conducted to look at the evidence of CBT used to treat tinnitus, hyperacusis, and misophonia.[94] As much as possible, they reviewed randomized controlled trials. They were able to find four published studies of CBT used to treat hyperacusis. Based on these four studies, the authors concluded, "the limited amount of available evidence supports the idea that CBT is effective in reducing hyperacusis handicap as measured via the Hyperacusis Questionnaire." (p. 998) (The Hyperacusis Questionnaire is described in appendix B.)

Another study evaluated the perspective of patients who had received audiologist-delivered CBT for their tinnitus and/or their hyperacusis.[102] The majority of 31 patients who completed a final survey following treatment felt that the CBT was "very acceptable" and "very effective."

Sound Therapy

A review of sound therapies for tinnitus and hyperacusis noted that these therapies are common.[74] It was observed that many patients reported their tinnitus became quieter or less bothersome, and that loud sounds became more tolerable. However, it was not clear if sound therapy was the reason for improvement or if it could be attributed to the counseling or to use of hearing aids. The author noted, "Clinical sound therapy trials are emerging, but outcomes typically remain modest, and few patients achieve complete remission of tinnitus or hyperacusis, unless the underlying hearing loss is treated with hearing aids or implants, in which case success rates are higher." [(p. 120)] In conclusion, the author stated, "Some tinnitus and hyperacusis patients respond remarkably well to sound therapy, whereas others don't benefit at all.... it appears that we've yet to reach sound therapy's full potential." [(p. 127)]

Another publication reviewed studies addressing the hypothesis that increased central auditory gain (see appendix F) is the mechanism underlying tinnitus and hyperacusis, and the effectiveness of treating these disorders with sound therapy.[75] They noted, "A large body of literature exists supporting the enhanced neural gain model of tinnitus and hyperacusis." [(p. 5)] They concluded, "The available literature from basic science studies supports the neural gain model of tinnitus and hyperacusis, which conceivably should be effectively managed with sound therapy." [(p. 5)]

Combined CBT and Sound Therapy

Few trials have been conducted to evaluate CBT for hyperacusis. Possibly the most rigorous of these trials involved six sessions of CBT over a two-month period.[95] Participants were instructed to use sound exposure in a controlled and stepwise fashion. Most of the outcome measures showed benefit for the CBT treatment group relative to a wait-list control group.

More recently, a study was conducted to evaluate treatment for hyperacusis "using sound exposure combined with breathing and relaxation strategies from both acceptance and commitment therapy and cognitive behavioral therapy."[96] [(p. 1)] All 30 of the patients had hyperacusis as their main complaint, and they received an average of six treatment sessions. Results were overall positive for reducing sensitivity to sound—both in the short term and the long term (six months).

Group Education

Investigators studied the approach of using a hyperacusis group educational session.[202] The session included explaining hyperacusis and its effects on daily life, the auditory system and how it relates to tinnitus and hyperacusis, and options for treatment. They concluded, "A group approach can facilitate the therapeutic process by connecting patients with others who are also affected by hyperacusis, and by educating patients and significant others on hyperacusis and its treatment options." [(p. 245)]

Surgery

A study was conducted to compare two "minimally invasive" surgeries to treat hyperacusis.[100] The surgeries involved reinforcing (stiffening) certain middle ear and inner ear structures. These structures included the round window, oval window, and stapes. The stapes is one of the three tiny middle ear bones that transmit sound from the eardrum to the cochlea (appendix E). The stapes pushes on the oval window to transmit sound to the fluid within the cochlea. The round window is like a "relief valve" for the cochlea—when the oval window is pushed in, the round window pushes out. The original surgical technique was round window reinforcement. The "new" technique added oval window and stapes reinforcement to the original technique. Comparing results, 80% of the patients receiving the new technique and 60% of those receiving the original technique showed improvement in hyperacusis symptoms. These results were sustained when patients were followed up an average of two years after surgery.

Migraine-Based Treatment

Appendix E contains a section describing how migraine can be associated with inner ear disorders, including loudness hyperacusis. A research group noted, "Hyperacusis as it relates to chronic migraine is well described."[97] (p. 2) They conducted a study with 25 hyperacusis patients to evaluate the efficacy of a "multi-modal prophylaxis therapy." The therapy consisted of dietary modifications (avoiding certain foods), dietary supplementation (magnesium and vitamin B2), eating three meals a day, sleeping on a regular schedule, and medications (prescribed in a stepwise manner). "The majority of patients with hyperacusis demonstrated symptomatic improvement.... as indicated by self-reported and audiometric measures." (p. 6)

Transitional Intervention

At the time of this writing, Transitional Intervention has been described in peer-reviewed publications for only a few months. The patented intervention (treatment) is specifically for loudness hyperacusis.[78] Why is it called "transitional"?

People with loudness hyperacusis naturally do whatever it takes to protect themselves from being exposed to sound that is uncomfortably loud. Those efforts involve some combination of wearing earplugs/earmuffs and avoiding being around the offending sound—protective behaviors that are reasonable and necessary to ensure comfort with sound in their environment. *Overdoing* these protective behaviors can, however, make the loudness hyperacusis worse. Why? Because overprotection deprives a person of normal exposure to sound. Sound deprivation can *increase central auditory gain*—meaning the brain's "volume control" is turned up, ultimately reducing the person's ability to tolerate the loudness of sounds.[26] (appendix A) The method is called "transitional" because the goal is to *transition* patients away from "their self-imposed silence.... to the starting point for acceptance and use of therapeutic sound in the treatment protocol."[87] (p. 1887)

Transitional intervention involves structured counseling, protective sound management, and therapeutic use of low-level broadband sound (sound therapy). The protocol "begins and ends with structured counseling."[78] Components of counseling include reviewing the patient's audiometric results; giving an overview of the transitional intervention protocol; describing the auditory system and the concept of central auditory gain; explaining how increased auditory gain can underlie loudness hyperacusis; explaining brain systems responsible for associated emotional reactions and stress; and the need to reduce the use of earplugs/earmuffs if they are overused.[87] All of this is background for counseling about how sound therapy can reduce auditory gain and lead to more normal functioning of the auditory system, and reduction or elimination of the associated reactions and stress. "As recalibration progresses, there will be less need for protected sound management and sound therapy. Sound tolerance will improve, hyperacusis will subside, and daily activities in typical healthy sound environments will again become routine."[87] (p. 1886)

The sound protection and sound therapy are accomplished with "protective treatment devices" (custom earpieces connected to behind-the-ear "intervention devices") that were specially developed for this protocol.[76] There are four objectives for their use: (1) provide controlled therapeutic (broadband) sound "to promote recalibration of the 'hypergain' processes that give rise to loudness hyperacusis"; (2) protect from uncomfortable sounds (using the custom earpieces that function as an earplug in isolation, and output-limited amplification—not exceeding comfortable levels—from the intervention devices); (3) gradually reduce the "misuse of hearing protection"; and (4) reduce sound-overprotection behaviors by gradually increasing amplification from the intervention devices.

A pilot study was conducted to evaluate "proof of concept" that people with "primary debilitating loudness hyperacusis can be successfully treated using the transitional intervention."[88] (p. 1904) Twelve participants completed the six-month protocol described above—structured counseling, protective sound management, and therapeutic sound. At each monthly visit, the output of the intervention devices was adjusted based on any changes in judgments of loudness when listening to running speech delivered from loudspeakers in a sound booth. The primary outcome measure was change in the output-limiting threshold for the devices. The mean change across participants was an increase of 35 dB. The authors concluded, "The outcomes from this trial were highly significant statistically and clinically based on sizable treatment-related change in the primary outcome measure.... and on meaningful change on those self-report questionnaires that addressed hyper-acusis- and sound-related problems and concerns of our participants." (p. 1918)

A series of four companion reports was published simultaneously to describe Transitional Intervention in detail: (1) background and rationale for the intervention;[78] (2) structured counseling;[87] (3) protective treatment devices;[76] and (4) field trial of the intervention.[88]

About the Author

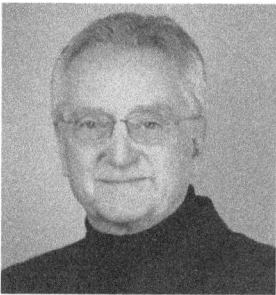

James A. Henry, PhD, is an audiologist with a doctorate in behavioral neuroscience. He spent over 35 years as an auditory researcher focusing mostly on tinnitus. During his career, he received funding of $28 million as principal or co-principal investigator for 43 projects and grants. He has authored over 250 publications, including more than 140 articles in peer-reviewed journals and eight books (this one is his ninth). He gave lectures and presentations nationally and internationally. His accomplishments resulted in numerous national awards.

Dr. Henry, who retired in 2022, continues to give lectures and training workshops, serves as an educational consultant, and has maintained his role as editor-at-large for the American Tinnitus Association's journal *Tinnitus Today*. His primary interest is writing books about tinnitus, sound hypersensitivity disorders, and hearing loss. This book is the fourth in a series under his corporation Ears Gone Wrong®, LLC.

The target audience for these books is both healthcare professionals and the lay public. The books are written with the rigor that is required for peer-reviewed journals, including hundreds of references to support the text. To make the books more accessible, technical and medical terms are minimized, and explained when used. Writing in this manner makes the books accessible to professionals in all healthcare disciplines as well as the general public.

Dr. Henry's website is www.earsgonewrong.org.

Acknowledgments

I am indebted to all of my former research and clinical colleagues from whom I learned so much. They are far too numerous to mention by name. I do, however, need to acknowledge Sarah Theodoroff, PhD, from whom I learned about noise sensitivity as a unique sound hypersensitivity disorder.

I have been fortunate to receive support and suggestions from Kelly Jahn, AuD, PhD and Hamid Djalilian, MD. Dr. Jahn answered questions about pain hyperacusis and provided me with numerous suggestions and important publications. Dr. Djalilian directly contributed to the sections in the book that address migraine and Ménière's disease. Drs. Jahn, Djalilian, and Theodoroff are greatly contributing to the advancement of the science pertaining to sound hypersensitivity disorders.

I've also learned from individuals who suffer from various forms of sound hypersensitivity. This book is dedicated to each and every one of them. I am especially grateful to David Treworgy, who informed me about pain hyperacusis and its devastating consequences. He wrote the insightful

Foreword to this book, which highlights the importance of why the book is needed. He also wrote a section in chapter 17 pertaining to available resources.

Significant edits were made by my wife, Mary Jo, who has a gift for making scientific language more accessible.

The book was proofread and copyedited by Robin L. Reed. Formatting of the book and book cover was done by Masha Shubin of Anno Domini Creative. Special thanks to both of them for their fine work.

References

1. Pienkowski M, Tyler RS, Roncancio ER, et al. A review of hyperacusis and future directions: Part II. Measurement, mechanisms, and treatment. *American Journal of Audiology.* 2014;23(4):420-36. doi:10.1044/2014_AJA-13-0037

2. Tyler RS, Pienkowski M, Roncancio ER, et al. A review of hyperacusis and future directions: part I. Definitions and manifestations. *American Journal of Audiology.* 2014;23(4):402-19. doi:10.1044/2014_AJA-14-0010

3. Williams ZJ, Suzman E, Woynaroski TG. A phenotypic comparison of loudness and pain hyperacusis: symptoms, comorbidity, and associated features in a multinational patient registry. *American Journal of Audiology.* 2021;30(2):341-358. doi:10.1044/2021_AJA-20-00209

4. Henry JA, Theodoroff SM, Edmonds C, et al. Sound tolerance conditions (hyperacusis, misophonia, noise sensitivity, and phonophobia): definitions and clinical management. *American Journal of Audiology*. 2022;31(3):513-527. doi:10.1044/2022_AJA-22-00035

5. Witt S. What I have learned from my hyperacusis patients. *Hearing Health Foundation (hearinghealth-foundation.org)*. 2023.

6. Treworgy D. My hope is to turn pain into progress. *Hearing Health*. 2023;39(2):30-33.

7. Wood MB, Nowak N, Fuchs PA. Damage-evoked signals in cochlear neurons and supporting cells. *Frontiers in Neurology*. 2024;15:1361747. doi:10.3389/fneur.2024.1361747

8. Palumbo DB, Alsalman O, De Ridder D, Song JJ, Vanneste S. Misophonia and potential underlying mechanisms: A perspective. *Frontiers in Psychology*. 2018;9:953. doi:10.3389/fpsyg.2018.00953

9. Fagelson M, Baguley DM. Disorders of sound tolerance: history and terminology. In: Fagelson M, Baguley DM, eds. *Hyperacusis and Disorders of Sound Intolerance: Clinical and Research Perspectives*. Plural Publishing, Inc.; 2018:3-14.

10. Siepsiak M, Dragan W. Misophonia - a review of research results and theoretical concepts. *Psychiatria Polska*. 2019;53(2):447-458. doi:10.12740/PP/92023

11. Shepherd D, Heinonen-Guzejev M, Hautus MJ, Heikkila K. Elucidating the relationship between noise sensitivity and personality. *Noise and Health*. 2015;17(76):165-71. doi:10.4103/1463-1741.155850

12. Asha'ari ZA, Mat Zain N, Razali A. Phonophobia and hyperacusis: practical points from a case report. *Malaysian Journal of Medical Sciences*. 2010;17(1):49-51.

13. Mor S, Grimaldos J, Tur C, et al. Internet- and mobile-based interventions for the treatment of specific phobia: A systematic review and preliminary meta-analysis. *Internet Interventions*. 2021;26:100462. doi:10.1016/j.invent.2021.100462

14. Lewine HE. Phobia. Harvard Health Publishing. Accessed December 20, 2024. https://www.health.harvard.edu/a_to_z/phobia-a-to-z

15. Fritscher L. Specific Phobia DSM-5 Diagnostic Criteria. Accessed December 20, 2024. https://www.verywell-mind.com/diagnosing-a-specific-phobia-2671981

16. Adams B, Sereda M, Casey A, Byrom P, Stockdale D, Hoare DJ. A Delphi survey to determine a definition and description of hyperacusis by clinician consensus. *International Journal of Audiology*. 2021;60(8):607-613. doi:10.1080/14992027.2020.1855370

17. Sherlock LP, Formby C. Considerations in the development of a sound tolerance interview and questionnaire instrument. *Seminars in Hearing*. 2017;38(1):53-70. doi:10.1055/s-0037-1598065

18. Formby C, Hawley ML, Sherlock LP, et al. A sound therapy-based intervention to expand the auditory dynamic range for loudness among persons with sensorineural hearing losses: A randomized placebo-controlled clinical trial. *Seminars in Hearing.* 2015;36(2):77-110. doi:10.1055/s-0035-1546958

19. Baguley DM, Hoare DJ. Hyperacusis: major research questions. *HNO.* 2018;66(5):358-363. doi:10.1007/s00106-017-0464-3

20. Anari M, Axelsson A, Eliasson A, Magnusson L. Hypersensitivity to sound--questionnaire data, audiometry and classification. *Scandinavian Audiology.* 1999;28(4):219-30. doi:10.1080/010503999424653

21. Filion PR, Margolis RH. Comparison of clinical and real-life judgments of loudness discomfort. *Journal of the American Academy of Audiology.* 1992;3(3):193-9.

22. Zaugg TL, Thielman EJ, Griest S, Henry JA. Subjective reports of trouble tolerating sound in daily life versus loudness discomfort levels. *American Journal of Audiology.* 2016;25(4):359-363. doi:10.1044/2016_AJA-15-0034

23. Dalkey NC. *The Delphi Method: An Experimental Study of Group Opinion. RM-5888-PR.* RAND Corporation; 1969.

24. Fackrell K, Potgieter I, Shekhawat GS, Baguley DM, Sereda M, Hoare DJ. Clinical interventions for hyperacusis in adults: a scoping review to assess the current position and determine priorities for research. *BioMed Research International.* 2017;2017:2723715. doi:10.1155/2017/2723715

25. McFerran D. Hyperacusis: medical diagnoses and associated syndromes. In: Fagelson M, Baguley DM, eds. *Hyperacusis and Disorders of Sound Intolerance: Clinical and Research Perspectives*. Plural Publishing, Inc.; 2018:107-131.

26. Henry JA. *The Tinnitus Book: Understanding Tinnitus and How To Find Relief.* Ears Gone Wrong, LLC; 2024.

27. Henry JA. *The Tinnitus Retraining Therapy Book: Walking You Through TRT*. Ears Gone Wrong, LLC; 2024.

28. Henry JA. *The Progressive Tinnitus Management Book: Step-by-Step Through the Five Levels of PTM*. Ears Gone Wrong, LLC; 2025.

29. Henry JA, Griest S, Zaugg TL, et al. Tinnitus and Hearing Survey: a screening tool to differentiate bothersome tinnitus from hearing difficulties. *American Journal of Audiology*. 2015;24(1):66-77. doi:10.1044/2014_AJA-14-0042

30. Henry JA, Zaugg TL, Myers PM, Kendall (Schmidt) CJ. *Progressive Tinnitus Management: Clinical Handbook for Audiologists*. Plural Publishing; 2010.

31. Grillon C. Models and mechanisms of anxiety: evidence from startle studies. *Psychopharmacology (Berl)*. 2008;199(3):421-37. doi:10.1007/s00213-007-1019-1

32. Evans RW, Seifert T, Kailasam J, Mathew NT. The use of questions to determine the presence of photophobia and phonophobia during migraine. *Headache*. 2008;48(3):395-7. doi:10.1111/j.1526-4610.2007.00920.x

33. Formby C, Sherlock LP, Gold SL. Adaptive plasticity of loudness induced by chronic attenuation and enhancement of the acoustic background. *Journal of the Acoustical Society of America*. 2003;114(1):55-8. doi:10.1121/1.1582860

34. Baguley DM, Andersson G. *Hyperacusis Mechanisms, Diagnosis, and Therapies*. Plural Publishing, Inc.; 2007.

35. Auerbach BD, Rodrigues PV, Salvi RJ. Central gain control in tinnitus and hyperacusis. *Frontiers in Neurology*. 2014;5:206. doi:10.3389/fneur.2014.00206

36. Schaette R, Kempter R. Development of tinnitus-related neuronal hyperactivity through homeostatic plasticity after hearing loss: a computational model. *European Journal of Neuroscience*. 2006;23(11):3124-38. doi:10.1111/j.1460-9568.2006.04774.x

37. Jahn KN, Kashiwagura ST, Yousuf MS. Clinical phenotype and management of sound-induced pain: Insights from adults with pain hyperacusis. *The Journal of Pain*. 27(104741):1-11. 2025. doi.org/10.1016/j.jpain.2024.104741

38. Cohen J. I have hyperacusis. Here's what it's like. *The Healthy Hearing Report (healthyhearing.com)*. November 28, 2022.

39. Liu C, Glowatzki E, Fuchs PA. Unmyelinated type II afferent neurons report cochlear damage. *Proceedings of the National Academy of Sciences*. Nov 24 2015;112(47):14723-7. doi:10.1073/pnas.1515228112

40. Flores EN, Duggan A, Madathany T, et al. A non-canonical pathway from cochlea to brain signals tissue-damaging noise. *Current Biology*. 2015;25(5):606-12. doi:10.1016/j.cub.2015.01.009

41. Tidball GA, Fagelson M. Audiological assessment of decreased sound tolerance. In: Fagelson M, Baguley DM, eds. *Hyperacusis and Disorders of Sound Intolerance*. Plural Publishing, Inc.; 2018:15-32.

42. Jastreboff MM, Jastreboff PJ. Decreased sound tolerance and Tinnitus Retraining Therapy (TRT). *Australian and New Zealand Journal of Audiology*. 2002;24:74-81.

43. Swedo SE, Baguley DM, Denys D, et al. Consensus definition of misophonia: A Delphi study. *Frontiers in Neuroscience*. 2022;16:841816. doi:10.3389/fnins.2022.841816

44. Paunovic KZ, Milenkovic SM. The proposed criteria for high perceived misophonia in young healthy adults and the association between misophonia symptoms and noise sensitivity. *Noise and Health*. 2022;24(113):40-48. doi:10.4103/nah.nah_40_20

45. Ferrer-Torres A, Gimenez-Llort L. Misophonia: A systematic review of current and future trends in this emerging clinical field. *International Journal of Environmental Research and Public Health*. 2022;19(11). doi:10.3390/ijerph19116790

46. Schroder A, Vulink N, Denys D. Misophonia: diagnostic criteria for a new psychiatric disorder. *PLoS One*. 2013;8(1):e54706. doi:10.1371/journal.pone.0054706

47. Bigras C, Theodoroff SM, Thielman EJ, Hebert S. Noise sensitivity or hyperacusis? Comparing the Weinstein and Khalfa questionnaires in a community and a clinical samples. *Hearing Research*. 2024;445:108992. doi:10.1016/j.heares.2024.108992

48. Stansfeld S, Clark C, Smuk M, Gallacher J, Babisch W. Road traffic noise, noise sensitivity, noise annoyance, psychological and physical health and mortality. *Environmental Health*. 2021;20(1):32. doi:10.1186/s12940-021-00720-3

49. Soto CJ, John OP. The next Big Five Inventory (BFI-2): Developing and assessing a hierarchical model with 15 facets to enhance bandwidth, fidelity, and predictive power. *Journal of Personality and Social Psychology*. 2017;113(1):117-143. doi:10.1037/pspp0000096

50. Shepherd D, Landon J, Kalloor M, Theadom A. Clinical correlates of noise sensitivity in patients with acute TBI. *Brain Injury*. 2019;33(8):1050-1058. doi:10.1080/02699052.2019.1606443

51. Zigmond AS, Snaith RP. The hospital anxiety and depression scale. *Acta Psychiatrica Scandinavica*. 1983;67(6):361-70. doi:10.1111/j.1600-0447.1983.tb09716.x

52. Park J, Chung S, Lee J, Sung JH, Cho SW, Sim CS. Noise sensitivity, rather than noise level, predicts the non-auditory effects of noise in community samples: a population-based survey. *BMC Public Health*. 2017;17(1):315. doi:10.1186/s12889-017-4244-5

53. Song C, Li H, Ma H, Han T, Wu J. Effects of noise type and noise sensitivity on working memory and noise annoyance. *Noise and Health*. 2022;24(114):173-181. doi:10.4103/nah.nah_6_22

54. Ghazavi Z, Davarinejad O, Jasimi F, Mohammadian Y, Sadeghi K. Noise sensitivity in patients with schizophrenia. *Noise and Health*. 2023;25(117):76-82. doi:10.4103/nah.nah_42_22

55. Welch D, Dirks KN, Shepherd D, Ong J. What is noise sensitivity? *Noise and Health*. 2022;24(114):158-165. doi:10.4103/nah.nah_56_21

56. Weinstein ND. Individual differences in reactions to noise: a longitudinal study in a college dormitory. *Journal of Applied Psychology*. 1978;63(4):458-66.

57. Schutte M, Marks A, Wenning E, Griefahn B. The development of the noise sensitivity questionnaire. *Noise and Health*. 2007;9(34):15-24. doi:10.4103/1463-1741.34700

58. Forbes D, Nickerson A, Bryant RA, et al. The impact of post-traumatic stress disorder symptomatology on quality of life: The sentinel experience of anger, hypervigilance and restricted affect. *Australian and New Zealand Journal of Psychiatry*. 2019;53(4):336-349. doi:10.1177/0004867418772917

59. Liberati AS, Perrotta G. Neuroanatomical and functional correlates in post-traumatic stress disorder: A narrative review. *Ibrain*. 2024;10(1):46-58. doi:10.1002/ibra.12147

60. Kliuchko M, Heinonen-Guzejev M, Vuust P, Tervaniemi M, Brattico E. A window into the brain mechanisms associated with noise sensitivity. *Scientific Reports*. 2016;6:39236. doi:10.1038/srep39236

61. Garcia R. Neurobiology of fear and specific phobias. *Learning and Memory*. 2017;24(9):462-471. doi:10.1101/lm.044115.116

62. American Psychiatric Association. Diagnostic and Statistical Manual of Mental Disorders, 5th ed. (2013).

63. Williams ZJ, Cascio CJ, Woynaroski TG. Psychometric validation of a brief self-report measure of misophonia symptoms and functional impairment: The Duke-Vanderbilt misophonia screening questionnaire. *Frontiers in Psychology*. 2022;13:897901. doi:10.3389/fpsyg.2022.897901

64. Williams ZJ, Suzman E, Woynaroski TG. Prevalence of decreased sound tolerance (hyperacusis) in individuals with autism spectrum disorder: a meta-analysis. *Ear and Hearing*. 2021;42(5):1137-1150. doi:10.1097/AUD.0000000000001005

65. LeDoux JE. The amygdala and emotion: A view through fear. In: Aggleton JP, ed. *The Amygdala: A Functional Analysis* Oxford University Press Inc.; 2000:289-310.

66. Iversen S, Kupfermann I, Kandel ER. Emotional states and feelings. In: Kandel ER, Schwartz JH, Jessell TM, eds. *Principles of Neural Science*. McGraw-Hill; 2000:982-997.

67. Eggermont JJ. Neuroplasticity of the auditory system. In: Schlee W, Langguth B, DeRidder D, Vanneste S, Kleinjung T, Møller AR, eds. *Textbook of Tinnitus*. 2nd ed. Springer; 2024:149-163.

68. McGill M, Hight AE, Watanabe YL, et al. Neural signatures of auditory hypersensitivity following acoustic trauma. *Elife*. 2022;11. doi:10.7554/eLife.80015

69. McFerran DJ, Baguley DM. Acoustic shock. *Journal of Laryngology and Otology*. 2007;121(4):301-5. doi:10.1017/S0022215107006111

70. Jacquemin L, Schecklmann M, Baguley DM. Hypersensitivity to sounds. In: Schlee W, Langguth B, DeRidder D, Vanneste S, Kleinjung T, Møller AR, eds. *Textbook of Tinnitus*. 2nd ed. Springer; 2024:25-34.

71. Noreña AJ, Fournier P, Londero A, Ponsot D, Charpentier N. An integrative model accounting for the symptom cluster triggered after an acoustic shock. *Trends in Hearing*. 2018;22:2331216518801725. doi:10.1177/2331216518801725

72. Fagelson M, Baguley DM, eds. *Hyperacusis and Disorders of Sound Intolerance: Clinical and Research Perspectives*. Plural Publishing; 2018.

73. Kalsoom N, Fackrell K, El Nsouli D, Carter H. Current recommendations for the use of sound therapy in adults with hyperacusis: a scoping review. *Brain Science*. 2024;14(8). doi:10.3390/brainsci14080797

74. Pienkowski M. Rationale and efficacy of sound therapies for tinnitus and hyperacusis. *Neuroscience*. 2019;407:120-134. doi:10.1016/j.neuroscience.2018.09.012

75. Sheppard A, Stocking C, Ralli M, Salvi R. A review of auditory gain, low-level noise and sound therapy for tinnitus and hyperacusis. *International Journal of Audiology*. 2020;59(1):5-15. doi:10.1080/14992027.2019.1660812

76. Eddins DA, Armstrong S, Juneau R, et al. Device and fitting protocol for a transitional intervention for debilitating hyperacusis. *Journal of Speech Language and Hearing Research*. 2024;67(6):1868-1885. doi:10.1044/2024_JSLHR-23-00359

77. Henry JA. Sound therapy to reduce auditory gain for hyperacusis and tinnitus. *American Journal of Audiology*. 2022;31(4):1067-1077. doi:10.1044/2022_AJA-22-00127

78. Formby C, Secor CA, Cherri D, Eddins DA. Background and rationale for a transitional intervention for debilitating hyperacusis. *Journal of Speech Language and Hearing Research*. 2024;67(6):1984-1993. doi:10.1044/2023_JSLHR-23-00352

79. Searchfield GD, Selvaratnam C. Hearing aids for decreased sound tolerance and minimal hearing loss: gain without pain. In: Fagelson M, Baguley DM, eds. *Hyperacusis and Disorders of Sound Intolerance: Clinical and Research Perspectives*. Plural Publishing, Inc.; 2018:223-239.

80. Vidal JL, Park JM, Han JS, Alshaikh H, Park SN. Measurement of loudness discomfort levels as a test for hyperacusis: test-retest reliability and its clinical value. *Clinical and Experimental Otorhinolaryngology.* 2022;15(1):84-90. doi:10.21053/ceo.2021.00318

81. Jastreboff PJ, Hazell JWP. *Tinnitus Retraining Therapy: Implementing the Neurophysiological Model.* Cambridge University Press; 2004.

82. Jastreboff PJ. Tinnitus Retraining Therapy. In: Møller AR, Langguth B, DeRidder D, Kleinjung T, eds. *Textbook of Tinnitus.* Springer; 2011:575-596.

83. Jastreboff PJ, Jastreboff MM. Tinnitus Retraining Therapy. In: Schlee W, Langguth B, DeRidder D, Vanneste S, Kleinjung T, Møller AR, eds. *Textbook of Tinnitus.* 2nd ed. Springer; 2024:589-616.

84. Tyler RS, Perreau A, Mancini PC. Hyperacusis. In: Tyler RS, Perreau A, eds. *Tinnitus Treatment: Clinical Protocols.* Thieme; 2022:165-197.

85. Perreau A, Tyler RS, Mancini PC, Witt SA. Tinnitus Activities Treatment. In: Tyler RS, Perreau A, eds. *Tinnitus Treatment: Clinical Protocols.* Thieme; 2022:42-70.

86. Henry JA, Zaugg TL, Myers PJ, Kendall (Schmidt) CJ. *Progressive Tinnitus Management: Counseling Guide.* Plural Publishing Inc; 2010.

87. Cherri D, Formby C, Secor CA, Eddins DA. Counseling protocol for a transitional intervention for debilitating hyperacusis. *Journal of Speech Language and Hearing Research*. 2024;67(6):1886-1902. doi:10.1044/2023_JSLHR-23-00353

88. Formby C, Cherri D, Secor CA, et al. Results of a 6-month field trial of a transitional intervention for debilitating hyperacusis. *Journal of Speech Language and Hearing Research*. 2024;67(6):1903-1931. doi:10.1044/2024_JSLHR-23-00360

89. Mehdi M, Dode A, Pryss R, Schlee W, Reichert M, Hauck FJ. Contemporary review of smartphone apps for tinnitus management and treatment. *Brain Sciences*. 2020;10(11). doi:10.3390/brainsci10110867

90. Cima RF, Andersson G, Schmidt CJ, Henry JA. Cognitive-behavioral treatments for tinnitus: a review of the literature. *Journal of the American Academy of Audiology*. 2014;25(1):29-61. doi:10.3766/jaaa.25.1.4

91. Fuller T, Cima R, Langguth B, Mazurek B, Vlaeyen JW, Hoare DJ. Cognitive Behavioural Therapy for tinnitus. *Cochrane Database Systematic Review*. 2020;1(1):CD012614. doi:10.1002/14651858.CD012614.pub2

92. Fuller TE, Haider HF, Kikidis D, et al. Different teams, same conclusions? A systematic review of existing clinical guidelines for the assessment and treatment of tinnitus in adults. *Frontiers in Psychology*. 2017;8:206. doi:10.3389/fpsyg.2017.00206

93. Tunkel DE, Bauer CA, Sun GH, et al. Clinical
     practice guideline: tinnitus. *Otolaryngology
     Head and Neck Surgery.* 2014;151(2 Suppl):S1-S40.
     doi:10.1177/0194599814545325

94. Aazh H, Landgrebe M, Danesh AA, Moore BC. Cog-
     nitive behavioral therapy for alleviating the distress
     caused by tinnitus, hyperacusis and misophonia: cur-
     rent perspectives. *Psychology Research and Behavior
     Management.* 2019;12:991-1002. doi:10.2147/PRBM.
     S179138

95. Juris L, Andersson G, Larsen HC, Ekselius L. Cogni-
     tive behaviour therapy for hyperacusis: a randomized
     controlled trial. *Behaviour Research and Therapy.*
     2014;54:30-7. doi:10.1016/j.brat.2014.01.001

96. Thieren S, van Dommelen P, Benard MR. New hyper-
     acusis therapy combines psychoeducation, sound
     exposure, and counseling. *American Journal of Audi-
     ology.* 2024:1-11. doi:10.1044/2024_AJA-23-00210

97. Abouzari M, Tan D, Sarna B, et al. Efficacy of multi-
     modal migraine prophylaxis therapy on hyperacusis
     patients. *Annals of Otology Rhinology and Laryngology.*
     2020;129(5):421-427. doi:10.1177/0003489419892997

98. Danesh AA, Howery S, Aazh H, Kaf W, Eshraghi AA.
     Hyperacusis in autism spectrum disorders. *Audi-
     ology Research.* 2021;11(4):547-556. doi:10.3390/
     audiolres11040049

99. Papesh MA, Theodoroff SM, Gallun FJ. Traumatic brain injury and auditory processing. In: Fagelson M, Baguley DM, eds. *Hyperacusis and Disorders of Sound Intolerance: Clinical and Research Perspectives.* Plural Publishing, Inc.; 2018:149-166.

100. Silverstein H, Kellermeyer B, Martinez U. Minimally invasive surgery for the treatment of hyperacusis: New technique and long term results. *American Journal of Otolaryngology.* 2020;41(1):102319. doi:10.1016/j.amjoto.2019.102319

101. Aazh H, Moore BCJ. Effectiveness of audiologist-delivered cognitive behavioral therapy for tinnitus and hyperacusis rehabilitation: outcomes for patients treated in routine practice. *American Journal of Audiology.* 2018;27(4):547-558. doi:10.1044/2018_AJA-17-0096

102. Aazh H, Bryant C, Moore BCJ. Patients' perspectives about the acceptability and effectiveness of audiologist-delivered cognitive behavioral therapy for tinnitus and/or hyperacusis rehabilitation. *American Journal of Audiology.* 2019;28(4):973-985. doi:10.1044/2019_AJA-19-0045

103. Henry JA, Goodworth MC, Lima E, Zaugg T, Thielman EJ. Cognitive behavioral therapy for tinnitus: Addressing the controversy of its clinical delivery by audiologists. *Ear and Hearing.* 2022;43(2):283-289. doi:10.1097/AUD.0000000000001150

104. Westcott M. Hyperacusis-induced pain: understanding and management of tonic tensor tympani syndrome (TTTS) symptoms. *Journal of Pain & Relief.* 2016;5(2):1-2. doi:10.4172/2167-0846.1000234

105. Fournier P, Paleressompoulle D, Esteve Fraysse MJ, et al. Exploring the middle ear function in patients with a cluster of symptoms including tinnitus, hyperacusis, ear fullness and/or pain. *Hearing Research*. 2022;422:108519. doi:10.1016/j.heares.2022.108519

106. Jastreboff PJ, Jastreboff MM. The neurophysiological approach to misophonia: Theory and treatment. *Frontiers in Neuroscience*. 2023;17:895574. doi:10.3389/fnins.2023.895574

107. Smith EEA, Guzick AG, Draper IA, et al. Perceptions of various treatment approaches for adults and children with misophonia. *Journal of Affective Disorders*. 2022;316:76-82. doi:10.1016/j.jad.2022.08.020

108. Mattson SA, D'Souza J, Wojcik KD, Guzick AG, Goodman WK, Storch EA. A systematic review of treatments for misophonia. *Precision Medicine in Psychiatry*. 2023;39-40. doi:10.1016/j.pmip.2023.100104

109. Jager IJ, Vulink NCC, Bergfeld IO, van Loon A, Denys D. Cognitive behavioral therapy for misophonia: A randomized clinical trial. *Depression Anxiety*. 2020;38(7):708-18. doi:10.1002/da.23127

110. Schroder AE, Vulink NC, van Loon AJ, Denys DA. Cognitive behavioral therapy is effective in misophonia: An open trial. *Journal of Affective Disorders*. 2017;217:289-294. doi:10.1016/j.jad.2017.04.017

111. Jastreboff PJ. The neurophysiological model of tinnitus and decreased sound tolerance. In: Schlee W, Langguth B, DeRidder D, Vanneste S, Kleinjung T, Møller AR, eds. *Textbook of Tinnitus*. 2nd ed. Springer; 2024:231-250.

112. Henry JA, Jastreboff MM, Jastreboff PJ, Schechter MA, Fausti SA. Guide to conducting Tinnitus Retraining Therapy initial and follow-up interviews. *Journal of Rehabilitation Research and Development*. 2003;40(2):157-77.

113. Henry JA, Trune DR, Robb MJA, Jastreboff PJ. *Tinnitus Retraining Therapy: Clinical Guidelines*. Plural Publishing, Inc.; 2007.

114. Jastreboff PJ, Jastreboff MM. Treatments for decreased sound tolerance (hyperacusis and misophonia). *Seminars in Hearing*. 2014;35(2):105-120. doi:10.1055/s-0034-1372527

115. Vanaja CS, Abigail MS. Misophonia: An evidence-based case report. *American Journal of Audiology*. 2020;29(4):685-690. doi:10.1044/2020_AJA-19-00111

116. Kamody RC, Del Conte GS. Using Dialectical Behavior Therapy to treat misophonia in adolescence. *Primary Care Companion for CNS Disorders*. 2017;19(5). doi:10.4088/PCC.17l02105

117. Schneider RL, Arch JJ. Case study: A novel application of mindfulness- and acceptance-based components to treat misophonia. *Journal of Contextual Behavioral Science*. 2017;6(2):221-225. doi:10.1016/j.jcbs.2017.04.003

118. Webb J, Williamson A. Steroids for the treatment of misophonia and misokinesia. *Case Reports in Psychiatry*. 2024;2024:3976837. doi:10.1155/2024/3976837

119. Natalini E, Fioretti A, Eibenstein R, Eibenstein A. Metacognitive interpersonal therapy for misophonia: A single-case study. *Brain Science*. 2024;14(7). doi:10.3390/brainsci14070717

120. Spencer SD, Mangen KH, Omar Y, Storch EA. Acceptance and Commitment Therapy for an emerging adult female with misophonia: A case study. *Journal of Psychiatric Practice*. 2024;30(5):374-378. doi:10.1097/PRA.0000000000000800

121. McMahon K, Cassiello-Robbins C, Greenleaf A, et al. The unified protocol for transdiagnostic treatment of emotional disorders for misophonia: a pilot trial exploring acceptability and efficacy. *Frontiers in Psychology*. 2023;14:1294571. doi:10.3389/fpsyg.2023.1294571

122. Qi L, Jilei Z, Lisheng Y, Yuanyuan J. Hyperacusis questionnaire and event-related potential correlation in migraine patients. *Scientific Reports*. 2024;14(1):14117. doi:10.1038/s41598-024-65014-3

123. Faulkner JW, Snell DL, Shepherd D, Theadom A. Turning away from sound: The role of fear avoidance in noise sensitivity following mild traumatic brain injury. *Journal of Psychosomatic Research*. 2021;151:110664. doi:10.1016/j.jpsychores.2021.110664

124. Landon J, Shepherd D, Stuart S, Theadom A, Freundlich S. Hearing every footstep: Noise sensitivity in individuals following traumatic brain injury. *Neuropsychological Rehabilitation*. 2012;22(3):391-407. doi:10.1080/09602011.2011.652496

125. Viziano A, Micarelli A, Alessandrini M. Noise sensitivity and hyperacusis in patients affected by multiple chemical sensitivity. *International Archives of Occupational and Environmental Health*. 2017;90(2):189-196. doi:10.1007/s00420-016-1185-8

126. Klein AJ, Armstrong BL, Greer MK, Brown FR, 3rd. Hyperacusis and otitis media in individuals with Williams syndrome. *Journal of Speech and Hearing Disorders*. 1990;55(2):339-44. doi:10.1044/jshd.5502.339

127. de Vries B, Leuven KU. Autism and the right to a hypersensitivity-friendly workspace. *Public Health Ethics*. 2021;14(3):281-287.

128. Theodoroff SM, Papesh M, Duffield T, et al. Concussion management guidelines neglect auditory symptoms. *Clinical Journal of Sport Medicine*. 2022;32(2):82-85. doi:10.1097/JSM.0000000000000874

129. Racz JI, Bialocerkowski A, Calteaux I, Farrell LJ. Determinants of exposure therapy implementation in clinical practice for the treatment of anxiety, OCD, and PTSD: A systematic review. *Clinical Child and Family Psychology Review*. 2024;27(2):317-341. doi:10.1007/s10567-024-00478-3

130. Kahl KG, Winter L, Schweiger U. The third wave of cognitive behavioural therapies: what is new and what is effective? *Current Opinions in Psychiatry.* 2012;25(6):522-8. doi:10.1097/YCO.0b013e328358e531

131. Rademaker MM, Stegeman I, Ho-Kang-You KE, Stokroos RJ, Smit AL. The effect of mindfulness-based interventions on tinnitus distress. A systematic review. *Frontiers in Neurology.* 2019;10:1135. doi:10.3389/fneur.2019.01135

132. Westin VZ, Schulin M, Hesser H, et al. Acceptance and Commitment Therapy versus Tinnitus Retraining Therapy in the treatment of tinnitus: a randomised controlled trial. *Behaviour Research and Therapy.* 2011;49(11):737-47. doi:10.1016/j.brat.2011.08.001

133. Hesser H, Gustafsson T, Lunden C, et al. A randomized controlled trial of Internet-delivered Cognitive Behavior Therapy and Acceptance and Commitment Therapy in the treatment of tinnitus. *Journal of Consulting and Clinical Psychology.* 2012;80(4):649-61. doi:10.1037/a0027021

134. Gans JJ, Holst J, Holmes C, Hudock D. Healing from home: Examination of an online mindfulness-based tinnitus stress reduction course during the 2020 COVID pandemic. *American Journal of Audiology.* 2023;32(1):160-169. doi:10.1044/2022_AJA-22-00063

135. Onyeka OC, Riddle D, Bivins E, et al. Internet-delivered cognitive behavioral therapy for anxiety. *Advances in Psychiatry and Behavioral Health.* 2024;4(1):91-100. doi:10.1016/j.ypsc.2024.05.003

136. Aazh H, Taylor L, Danesh AA, Moore BCJ. The effectiveness of unguided internet-based cognitive behavioral therapy for tinnitus for patients with tinnitus alone or combined with hyperacusis and/or misophonia: a preliminary analysis. *Journal of the American Academy of Audiology.* 2022;33(7-08):405-416. doi:10.1055/a-2087-0262

137. Mueller HG, Bentler RA. Fitting hearing aids using clinical measures of loudness discomfort levels: an evidence-based review of effectiveness. *Journal of the American Academy of Audiology.* 2005;16(7):461-72. doi:10.3766/jaaa.16.7.6

138. Jastreboff PJ, Hazell JW. A neurophysiological approach to tinnitus: clinical implications. *British Journal of Audiology.* 1993;27(1):7-17. doi:10.3109/03005369309077884

139. Khalfa S, Dubal S, Veuillet E, Perez-Diaz F, Jouvent R, Collet L. Psychometric normalization of a hyperacusis questionnaire. *ORL Journal of Otorhinolaryngology and Related Specialties.* 2002;64(6):436-42. doi:10.1159/000067570

140. Fackrell K, Fearnley C, Hoare DJ, Sereda M. Hyperacusis Questionnaire as a tool for measuring hypersensitivity to sound in a tinnitus research population. *BioMed Research International.* 2015;2015:290425. doi:10.1155/2015/290425

141. Nelting M, Rienhoff NK, Hesse G, Lamparter U. [The assessment of subjective distress related to hyperacusis with a self-rating questionnaire on hypersensitivity to sound]. *Laryngorhinootologie.* 2002;81(5):327-34. doi:10.1055/s-2002-28342

142. Blasing L, Goebel G, Flotzinger U, Berthold A, Kroner-Herwig B. Hypersensitivity to sound in tinnitus patients: an analysis of a construct based on questionnaire and audiological data. *International Journal of Audiology*. 2010;49(7):518-26. doi:10.3109/14992021003724996

143. Dauman R, Bouscau-Faure F. Assessment and amelioration of hyperacusis in tinnitus patients. *Acta Otolaryngologica*. 2005;125(5):503-9. doi:10.1080/00016480510027565

144. Greenberg B, Carlos M. Psychometric properties and factor structure of a new scale to measure hyperacusis: Introducing the Inventory of Hyperacusis Symptoms. *Ear and Hearing*. 2018;39(5):1025-1034. doi:10.1097/AUD.0000000000000583

145. Aazh H, Danesh AA, Moore BCJ. Internal consistency and convergent validity of the Inventory of Hyperacusis Symptoms. *Ear and Hearing*. 2021;42(4):917-926. doi:10.1097/AUD.0000000000000982

146. Prabhu P, Nagaraj MK. Development and validation of Hyperacusis Handicap Questionnaire in individuals with tinnitus associated with hyperacusis. *Journal of Otology*. 2020;15(4):124-128. doi:10.1016/j.joto.2019.12.004

147. Aazh H, Hayes C, Moore BCJ, Danesh AA, Vitoratou S. Psychometric evaluation of the Hyperacusis Impact Questionnaire (HIQ) and Sound Sensitivity Symptoms Questionnaire (SSSQ) using a clinical population of adult patients with tinnitus alone or combined with hyperacusis. *Journal of the American Academy of Audiology*. 2022;33(5):248-258. doi:10.1055/a-1780-4002

148. Raj-Koziak D, Gos E, Kutyba JJ, Skarzynski PH, Skarzynski H. Hyperacusis Assessment Questionnaire-A new tool assessing hyperacusis in subjects with tinnitus. *Journal of Clinical Medicine*. 2023;12(20). doi:10.3390/jcm12206622

149. Goodman WK, Price LH, Rasmussen SA, et al. The Yale-Brown Obsessive Compulsive Scale. I. Development, use, and reliability. *Archives of General Psychiatry*. 1989;46(11):1006-11. doi:10.1001/archpsyc.1989.01810110048007

150. Goodman WK, Price LH, Rasmussen SA, et al. The Yale-Brown Obsessive Compulsive Scale. II. Validity. *Archives of General Psychiatry*. 1989;46(11):1012-6. doi:10.1001/archpsyc.1989.01810110054008

151. Yektatalab S, Mohammadi A, Zarshenas L. The prevalence of misophonia and its relationship with obsessive-compulsive disorder, anxiety, and depression in undergraduate students of Shiraz University of Medical Sciences: a cross-sectional study. *International Journal of Community Based Nurssing and Midwifery*. 2022;10(4):259-268. doi:10.30476/IJCBNM.2022.92902.1888

152. Rosenthal MZ, Anand D, Cassiello-Robbins C, et al. Development and initial validation of the Duke Misophonia Questionnaire. *Frontiers in Psychology.* 2021;12:709928. doi:10.3389/fpsyg.2021.709928

153. Wu MS, Lewin AB, Murphy TK, Storch EA. Misophonia: incidence, phenomenology, and clinical correlates in an undergraduate student sample. *Journal of Clinical Psychology.* 2014;70(10):994-1007. doi:10.1002/jclp.22098

154. Dibb B, Golding SE, Dozier TH. The development and validation of the Misophonia response scale. *Journal of Psychosomatic Research.* 2021;149:110587. doi:10.1016/j.jpsychores.2021.110587

155. Siepsiak M, Sliwerski A, Lukasz Dragan W. Development and psychometric properties of MisoQuest-A new self-report questionnaire for misophonia. *International Journal of Environmental Research and Public Health.* 2020;17(5). doi:10.3390/ijerph17051797

156. Jager I, de Koning P, Bost T, Denys D, Vulink N. Misophonia: Phenomenology, comorbidity and demographics in a large sample. *PLoS One.* 2020;15(4):e0231390. doi:10.1371/journal.pone.0231390

157. Worthington DL, Bodie G, eds. *The Sourcebook of Listening Research: Methodology and Measures.* John Wiley & Sons, Inc.; 2018.

158. Shepherd D, Hautus MJ, Lee SY, Mulgrew J. Electrophysiological approaches to noise sensitivity. *Journal of Clinical and Experimental Neuropsychology.* 2016;38(8):900-12. doi:10.1080/13803395.2016.1176995

159. Blaesing L, Kroener-Herwig B. Self-reported and behavioral sound avoidance in tinnitus and hyperacusis subjects, and association with anxiety ratings. *International Journal of Audiology*. 2012;51(8):611-7. doi: 10.3109/14992027.2012.664290

160. Lebeau RT, Glenn DE, Hanover LN, Beesdo-Baum K, Wittchen HU, Craske MG. A dimensional approach to measuring anxiety for DSM-5. *International Journal of Methods in Psychiatric Research*. 2012;21(4):258-72. doi:10.1002/mpr.1369

161. Cederroth CR, Lugo A, Edvall NK, et al. Association between hyperacusis and tinnitus. *Journal of Clinical Medicine*. 2020;9(8). doi:10.3390/jcm9082412

162. Hiller W, Goebel G. When tinnitus loudness and annoyance are discrepant: audiological characteristics and psychological profile. *Audiology and Neurootology*. 2007;12(6):391-400. doi:10.1159/000106482

163. Guan X, Cheng YS, Galaiya DJ, Rosowski JJ, Lee DJ, Nakajima HH. Bone-conduction hyperacusis induced by superior canal dehiscence in human: the underlying mechanism. *Scientific Reports*. 2020;10(1):16564. doi:10.1038/s41598-020-73565-4

164. Edmonson A, Iwanaga J, Olewnik L, Dumont AS, Tubbs RS. The function of the tensor tympani muscle: a comprehensive review of the literature. *Anatomy & Cell Biology*. 2022;55(2):113-117. doi:10.5115/acb.21.032

165. Jones SE, Mason MJ, Sunkaraneni VS, Baguley DM. The effect of auditory stimulation on the tensor tympani in patients following stapedectomy. *Acta Otolaryngologica*. 2008;128(3):250-4. doi:10.1080/00016480701509925

166. Littwin R. Hyperacusis management: a patient's perspective. In: Fagelson M, Baguley DM, eds. *Hyperacusis and Disorders of Sound Intolerance*. Plural Publishing, Inc.; 2018:241-263.

167. Schaette R. Peripheral mechanisms of decreased sound tolerance. In: Fagelson M, Baguley DM, eds. *Hyperacusis and Disorders of Sound Intolerance: Clinical and Research Perspectives*. Plural Publishing, Inc.; 2018:61-75.

168. Saxena U, Singh BP, Kumar SBR, Chacko G, Bharath K. Acoustic reflexes in individuals having hyperacusis of the auditory origin. *Indian Journal of Otolaryngology Head & Neck Surgery*. 2020;72(4):497-502. doi:10.1007/s12070-020-02002-9

169. Møller AR. Neurophysiological basis of the acoustic middle-ear reflex. In: Silman S, ed. *The Acoustic Reflex: Basic Principles and Clinical Applications*. Academic Press, Inc.; 1984:1-34.

170. Westcott M, Sanchez TG, Diges I, et al. Tonic tensor tympani syndrome in tinnitus and hyperacusis patients: a multi-clinic prevalence study. *Noise and Health*. 2013;15(63):117-28. doi:10.4103/1463-1741.110295

171. Klockhoff, I. Impedance fluctuation and a 'tensor tympani syndrome.' Proceedings of the 4th International Symposium on Acoustic Impedance Measurements, Lisbon. 1979:69-76.

172. Henry JA, Djalilian H. Navigating the complexities of migraine, Ménière's disease, tinnitus, and hyperacusis. *Tinnitus Today*. 2024;49(3):51-55.

173. Umemoto KK, Tawk K, Mazhari N, Abouzari M, Djalilian HR. Management of migraine-associated vestibulocochlear disorders. *Audiology Research*. 2023;13(4):528-545. doi:10.3390/audiolres13040047

174. Vingen JV, Sand T, Stovner LJ. Sensitivity to various stimuli in primary headaches: a questionnaire study. *Headache*. 1999;39(8):552-8. doi:10.1046/j.1526-4610.1999.3908552.x

175. Ahmad JG, Lin KF. Ménière's disease is a disorder of the inner ear. *Current Opinion in Otolaryngology & Head and Neck Surgery*. 2023;31(5):320-324. doi:10.1097/MOO.0000000000000921

176. Sarna B, Abouzari M, Lin HW, Djalilian HR. A hypothetical proposal for association between migraine and Ménière's disease. *Medical Hypotheses*. 2020;134:109430. doi:10.1016/j.mehy.2019.109430

177. Frank M, Abouzari M, Djalilian HR. Ménière's disease is a manifestation of migraine. *Current Opinion in Otolaryngology & Head and Neck Surgery*. 2023;31(5):313-319. doi:10.1097/MOO.0000000000000908

178. Ghavami Y, Mahboubi H, Yau AY, Maducdoc M, Djalilian HR. Migraine features in patients with Ménière's disease. *Laryngoscope.* 2016;126(1):163-8. doi:10.1002/lary.25344

179. Moshtaghi O, Sahyouni R, Lin HW, Ghavami Y, Djalilian HR. A historical recount: discovering Ménière's disease and its association with migraine headaches. *Otology and Neurotology.* 2016;37(8):1199-203. doi:10.1097/MAO.0000000000001122

180. Zagolski O, Papiez P, Kruk B, Kruk D. Tinnitus characteristics in patients with hyperacusis and vertigo (including Ménière's disease) vs. hyperacusis alone. *Acta Otorrinolaringologica (English Edition).* 2023;74(1):8-14. doi:10.1016/j.otoeng.2021.09.004

181. Beh SC, Masrour S, Smith SV, Friedman DI. The spectrum of vestibular migraine: clinical features, triggers, and examination findings. *Headache.* 2019;59(5):727-740. doi:10.1111/head.13484

182. Jones C. Glasgow Coma Scale. *American Journal Of Nursing.* 1979;79(9):1551-3.

183. Ray S, Luke J, Kreitzer N. Patient-centered mild traumatic brain injury interventions in the emergency department. *The American Journal of Emergency Medicine.* 2024;79:183-191. doi:10.1016/j.ajem.2024.02.038

184. Assi H, Moore RD, Ellemberg D, Hebert S. Sensitivity to sounds in sport-related concussed athletes: a new clinical presentation of hyperacusis. *Scientific Reports.* 2018;8(1):9921. doi:10.1038/s41598-018-28312-1

185. Weber H, Pfadenhauer K, Stohr M, Rosler A. Central hyperacusis with phonophobia in multiple sclerosis. *Multiple Sclerosis*. 2002;8(6):505-9. doi:10.1191/1352458502ms814oa

186. Thabet EM, Zaghloul HS. Auditory profile and high resolution CT scan in autism spectrum disorders children with auditory hypersensitivity. *European Archives of Otorhinolaryngology*. 2013;270(8):2353-8. doi:10.1007/s00405-013-2482-4

187. Lukose R, Brown K, Barber CM, Kulesza RJ, Jr. Quantification of the stapedial reflex reveals delayed responses in autism. *Autism Research*. 2013;6(5):344-53. doi:10.1002/aur.1297

188. Fagelson MA. The association between tinnitus and posttraumatic stress disorder. *American Journal of Audiology*. 2007;16(2):107-17. doi:10.1044/1059-0889(2007/015)

189. Paulin J, Andersson L, Nordin S. Characteristics of hyperacusis in the general population. *Noise and Health*. 2016;18(83):178-84. doi:10.4103/1463-1741.189244

190. Auerbach BD, Gritton HJ. Hearing in complex environments: Auditory gain control, attention, and hearing loss. *Frontiers in Neuroscience*. 2022;16:799787. doi:10.3389/fnins.2022.799787

191. Dubin AE, Patapoutian A. Nociceptors: the sensors of the pain pathway. *Journal of Clinical Investigation*. 2010;120(11):3760-72. doi:10.1172/JCI42843

192. Arcilla CK, Tadi P. Neuroanatomy, Unmyelinated Nerve Fibers. *StatPearls*. 2024.

193. Henry JA, Thielman EJ, Zaugg T, Griest S, Stewart BJ. Assessing meaningful improvement: focus on the Tinnitus Functional Index. *Ear and Hearing*. 2024;45(3):537-549. doi:10.1097/AUD.0000000000001456

194. Wood MB. Understanding pain signals triggered by damage to the inner ear. Hearing Health Foundation. April 3, 2024. hearinghealthfoundation.org

195. Goldberg LR. An alternative "description of personality": the big-five factor structure. *Journal of Personality and Social Psychology*. 1990;59(6):1216-29. doi:10.1037//0022-3514.59.6.1216

196. Durai M, Searchfield G. Anxiety and depression, personality traits relevant to tinnitus: A scoping review. *International Journal of Audiology*. 2016;55(11):605-15. doi:10.1080/14992027.2016.1198966

197. Bartels H, Middel BL, van der Laan BF, Staal MJ, Albers FW. The additive effect of co-occurring anxiety and depression on health status, quality of life and coping strategies in help-seeking tinnitus sufferers. *Ear and Hearing*. 2008;29(6):947-56. doi:10.1097/AUD.0b013e3181888f83

198. Strumila R, Lengvenyte A, Vainutiene V, Lesinskas E. The role of questioning environment, personality traits, depressive and anxiety symptoms in tinnitus severity perception. *Psychiatry Quarterly*. 2017;88(4):865-877. doi:10.1007/s11126-017-9502-2

199. Heinonen-Guzejev M, Vuorinen HS, Mussalo-Rauhamaa H, Heikkila K, Koskenvuo M, Kaprio J. Genetic component of noise sensitivity. *Twin Research and Human Genetics*. 2005;8(3):245-9. doi:10.1375/1832427054253112

200. Park JM, Kim WJ, Ha JB, Han JJ, Park SY, Park SN. Effect of sound generator on tinnitus and hyperacusis. *Acta Otolaryngologica*. 2018;138(2):135-139. doi:10.1080/00016489.2017.1386801

201. Aazh H, Knipper M, Danesh AA, et al. Insights from the third international conference on hyperacusis: causes, evaluation, diagnosis, and treatment. *Noise & Health*. 2018;20(95):162-170. doi:10.4103/nah.NAH_2_18

202. Perreau AE, Tyler RS, Mancini PC, Witt S, Elgandy MS. Establishing a group educational session for hyperacusis patients. *American Journal of Audiology*. 2019;28(2):245-250. doi:10.1044/2019_AJA-18-0148

Index